Awaken Your Wellbeing

Transformational Stories of Courage, Hope, and Healing

All proceeds of this book go to Galway Simon Community to prevent homelessness

Orla Kelly Publishing
Kilbrody, Mount Oval
Rochestown, Cork
Ireland.

Disclaimer

This book has been written for self-care and educational purposes. It does not offer any guarantees and assumes no liability of any kind in respect of the accuracy or completeness of its contents. The authors shall not be held liable or responsible to any person or entity with regard to issues of mental, physical or general health or wellbeing. Nor to any consequential physical, mental or general health issues alleged to have been caused directly or indirectly by the information or content of this book.

Contents

Intention Of This Book

If there is one thing I would like you to take from this book, it is this: *To Help You Help Yourself.*

In 2018, I published my first book '*Someone please help me, So I did*' in which I shared with my readers the story of how from my childhood experiences of sexual abuse, it led me to an existence of anxiety, depression and suicidal thoughts. In the book, I shared my vulnerability and my deepest truths in the hope that it would help others to help themselves.

I shared with readers how I learned from the darkest times in my life that I had to choose to help myself if I wanted to survive firstly, but also to then thrive. I shared how I found different wellbeing tools and techniques that helped me heal on all levels – physical, mental, emotional, and spiritual.

It was a daily choice and one that led me to train in different therapies that would help myself firstly and lead me to this very moment secondly, and ultimately, to the work I am now doing with so many people around the world.

I was overwhelmed with the response to my book, in that, so many people contacted me after reading it and told me it was their story too. They all wanted to know "Where do I start?" and it got me thinking about how not one size fits all and that we each have to find ways that resonate with us in each moment and each part of our healing or wellbeing.

I had so many requests to speak at different events and I knew that I wanted to reach more people and help them find a way to know that there is so much support out there, if they just took that one step in reaching out and asking for help. And from that thought, this book manifested as I reached out and invited the wonderful people who are in it to share their experiences with all of you. They too have been through many life challenges and have learned ways not only to help themselves but now like me, are helping others. They have a wealth of experience in their own chosen fields and through reading each chapter, you will gain a deeper understanding and awareness of how each therapy works and if it is right for you.

In this book, we are a collaboration of energy and wisdom. We share with you the experiences that have brought us to this point in our lives, in the way that our struggles have shaped the people we are today, but along the way, we have learned to open up the door of our hearts and minds to *awaken our wellbeing* to reach our highest potential. We are still learning but are open and willing to doing so.

Together we are stronger and in sharing this book with you, we hope that it will give you the strength and courage to reach your full potential. We all have bad days, but that is not a way to describe your whole life. We learn from the challenges and bring forth the lessons we learn from them in a new and positive way.

We learn that we cannot control every situation around us, but that we can control how we react to them. We learn that in the saddest of times, we can still feel joy. We learn that in the toughest of struggles, there is still hope. We learn that when we give up hope, we are giving up on ourselves.

We want to help you find a way back on your path and in which you will find your own direction.

This book is a testimony to life and that we all deserve the best life possible, but first we must believe that it is possible, I believe it is.

I want to thank all the contributors of this book for their generosity of spirit and knowledge. Together and with your support, we are hoping to make a difference, not only to the readers but also the people who are supported and cared for through the tireless work of Galway Simon Community in preventing homelessness.

Sharon Fitzmaurice

Introduction

Welcome to *Awaken Your Wellbeing*. Wellbeing is defined as a state of wellness in which every person realises their own potential; they can cope with normal stresses of life and are able to contribute to their own life, to their families, their communities, and the world.

But what if life stresses become too much? How do we find the resources within ourselves to manage, cope or heal that which we cannot seem to find a solution to?

Firstly, it is acknowledging you have a problem.

Secondly, it is accepting that you need support.

Thirdly, it is allowing yourself to explore all options.

When you are aware that you have options, it takes the huge fear out of the problem and you can take that next step to finding a solution that works for you as an individual.

In this book, we work on the ethos of treating the whole self — mind, body and spirit. This is known as a holistic approach.

We do not just treat the symptoms — we treat the whole person. Every part of your body works together, and each part influences the other. Our mind and emotions affect our body.

The word holistic comes from the Greek word *holos* meaning 'entire' or 'all.' A holistic view is that all aspects of peoples needs, psychological, physical, and social, should be considered when treating them.

We as human beings are unique, but we will at some point in our lives experience an imbalance whether it be physically, mentally, emotionally, or spiritually. The holistic approach is there to help achieve balance in all areas.

When we take a holistic approach, we look at the whole person and try to learn the underlying cause of an issue. We work together to help you to help yourself and find out what is causing the imbalance. The client and the therapist work together.

You do not have to be sick or unwell to benefit from a holistic approach to wellbeing as it encompasses all aspects of life.

In this book, we share with our readers the knowledge we have gained from our training and experience to help you gain a better understanding of how the mind affects the body, how our environment socially and emotionally has an effect on our behaviours, patterns and beliefs and how you all have the potential within you to be well.

We will share with you our client's stories and how they made a choice to make a change within their own lives. When we are informed, we have the power to make better choices.

To reach our greatest potential, we sometimes must face our greatest fears.

Foreword from Galway Simon Community

It can be difficult to understand the impact that homelessness can have on a person. Not having a safe place to call home, or the security of one's own front door can have a profound effect on a person's emotional and mental health. Anxiety and uncertainty dominate. Some become overwhelmed, some become stoic, some become profoundly distressed. What has to be remembered about Ireland today is that people of all ages can and do become homeless. Within our services we meet people facing homelessness for the first time in their lives at the point of retirement, and we are also working with families where children are being born into homelessness.

We in Galway Simon Community remain committed to the people who are most affected by homelessness. We provide a range of services, including accommodation with intensive support to those who have been chronically homeless for long periods of their lives, as well as Community Prevention Services that seek to co-ordinate solutions to ensure that individuals and families can avoid emergency homelessness. We strive to be effective and solution focused to help people solve their immediate problem and we also offer comprehensive supports to people to make realistic plans for their medium and long term future.

We get to make a real difference to many people on an ongoing basis, and we manage to do this because we harness the support of the wider community to enable us to carry out our work. The true concern, compassion and solidarity of people is so critical to our work and our effectiveness, and our clients are very often sustained by this.

We are particularly grateful to Sharon Fitzmaurice for her ongoing support, and we are deeply thankful to her and her fellow co-authors for so generously donating the proceeds their *Awaken Your Wellbeing* book to Galway Simon Community. We also wish to express our gratitude to all of those who purchase this book for the support they are providing to our clients. With your continued support, we will be able to offer our services to those who need us when they are most vulnerable.

Karen Feeney
Head of Client Services

My Breakdown Was My Breakthrough
by Marian Trench

My name is Marian Trench and I am from a little village in County Roscommon in the west of Ireland. I am forty-eight years of age, married to John and we have two children together whom we adore. At the time of writing, Ava is twenty years old and Jack is seventeen.

Why am I involved in this book?

I will give you an in-depth look at my journey and explain where I am coming from. I hope that my story will enlighten any individuals going forward on why I used Energy Healing as a modality for my recovery.

I was born in Galway on the 21st of May 1972, weighing over eleven pounds – no doubt causing huge difficulty for my poor mother. I was reared in a middle-class home and lived with my parents, two older brothers and one younger sister. From my entrance to this world, life presented challenges for my family and in turn, I am sure my parents coping mechanisms were autonomic as I began to deal with life and the journey it presented to me.

The trauma of my delivery and birth would have made an immediate impact on my system. My mother was two days in labour with me, thus causing enormous stress for me, the baby and undoubtedly huge pain, anguish, and anger for my mother in delivery.

Fast forward to six months of age, there was a huge house fire and our home was completely gutted and everything my parents had was destroyed. They had no money, no home, no house insurance. As a baby, I had unconsciously absorbed all their stresses, anxieties, and pain.

We moved back with my grandparents until such time my parents had our new home ready and we could all return to being one big happy family. I had grown to love my grandparents and loved staying with them, and for months at a time, I would live there. I felt safe, loved, and nurtured. As the years went by, I constantly had kidney infections and was hospitalised for weeks at a time. Back then you might have visitors once in a blue moon and my mother may write a note, then post it to me as a way of staying in touch as there wouldn't have phone contact, transport, etc. How alien does that seem in comparison to nowadays?

As I grew up, I had learnt different skills in how to earn love, respect, and acceptance. This varied from keeping quiet, hard work and eating everything that was put in front of me – shut up, put up and eat up. Life events left me scarred. I was living in survival mode and didn't realise the impact of such a huge scar on my young brain, body, and soul and I am sure neither did my parents. This is not about blaming anyone nor pointing the finger; it is just the reality of my home life and no doubt the homes of many, many more at the time. When we know better, we do better or at least, we try.

I was now coming into my pre-teens and had learnt how to keep secrets to survive. I developed mechanisms for carrying other people's problems. I was full of insecurities, and my vision was not great. I was overweight and did not feel like I fitted in. I genuinely thought that I was not pretty and I had all the insecurities any teenager would have these days of not being enough or not doing enough to please someone else. All of the above were my reality as I continued into secondary school. My shyness was at its peak, and my anxiety continued (even though I did not know what it was). I wanted to be as cool as the girl beside me, I wanted to be as smart as the other girl beside me, I wanted to be as fast as the other team members on the basketball court, I wanted it all, but I was not feeling it.

I knew what I had to do, work harder, go on a diet, fit in – all of which were my survival instincts from a young age. None of my insecurities derived from any member in secondary school; they had happened long before then, but different events in secondary school compounded the anxieties I had already developed.

Turning sixteen/seventeen, I was coming into an age of beginning to know myself, or was I? I had gone on a rapid summer holiday diet, and had lost three or four stone in weight. No one recognised me on my return to school. I was borderline anorexic. Teachers were concerned, my parents were concerned, my sister was concerned. However, I felt I was still not 'enough'. I was nearing my late teens, yet I had never had my period. This was a huge concern for my mother. To me at that time, it was a case of 'So what!' Talking about that area of my body was a big no. My mother, thankfully, took me to a new doctor in the town at the time. Dr Jarlath was approachable and professional and to this day he remains the same. Thank you Dr Jarlath. Straight away, he was concerned and within a week, I was hospitalised. I had surgery and an ovarian cyst was removed. I was quite sick for a few days after surgery.

Events from my past started coming to my mind, but I had no idea all of this was reflective on my body, mind, or its wellbeing. The following week I had received my first period and have never looked back apart from the odd irregular cycle. Doctors told my mother at that time that I may never conceive, but she managed to keep this to herself. To be honest, I am thankful as I do believe it may have planted a negative thought and possibly the conception of our two beautiful children might not have happened.

My 'physical' body recovered, and I continued my schooling and did my Leaving Cert. Again there was huge anxiety around this time of my life as 'not enough' thoughts were creeping into me or rather was part of me and was autonomic. I did well as I was 'intellectually savvy' but 'emotionally vulnerable/weak'. No one considered emotions as part of our wellbeing back then. Everything was hidden, not discussed openly and secrets were centrefold.

That summer, I applied for a secretarial position within a local busy insurance brokerage and was successful. Little did I think that twenty years on, I would have still be an employee. Time went on, and I had met so many people in the insurance business, some of whom I am still in contact and remain exceptionally good friends with. I met my husband John and married a few years later. Fast forward six months after our marriage, our lives changed forever. We were involved in a farm accident at our home where John's nephew was killed instantly in a tractor accident. We were young, and we had no idea of life and we had no idea of the support that was available to us. We lived in fear, we lived in anger, we lived with all the 'what ifs'. Together, we never spoke about the "accident", but to others, we would have been more open. Looking back, I think it was our fear of bringing it up as it was going to hurt both of us.

A few weeks after the accident, we both returned to work and continued with our lives as best as we possibly could or at least that is what we thought. Shortly after, our little girl was born prematurely. I am now more consciously aware that the stress carried by the mother in pregnancy can and most naturally will be transferred to the baby. My goodness did Ava cry. We paced the floors, roads, you name it and following years of antibiotics, my husband begged me to bring her to a "Bio Energy Therapist". I feared that it was whacky and would do my daughter more harm than good. However, after the first session was the first night sleep myself and John had in years. I believe Ava's crying was initiated by her mother's pain (my pain), but I was ignorant to this back then. Following two years and ten months after Ava's birth, our little boy Jack Trench was born. He appeared more relaxed and at ease. Some might say like an old man sitting at a bar, just chilled and content.

A few weeks after Jack's birth, John developed Viral Meningitis. The following year, my best friend's husband was killed in a car crash and a couple of years later, Jack was tested for Leukaemia following a fall and an injury that led to a small bleed. All tests were clear, thank God but I had lived in constant fear that something terrible was going to happen of something happening to my children.

We worked extremely hard, thinking we were making a better future for them; when in fact, we were paying somebody to rear our children, our biggest pride and joy and missing out on this time with them. Yes, I do know that both parents nowadays may need to work outside the home to make ends meet but believe me, I didn't know where to stop until one day, following various 'anxiety attacks', I had no other choice but to seek help. I was rushing, getting the kids ready for the babysitter, for playschool and then trying to arrive at work on time. I had been reading a book called *The Secret*. I was addicted to reading it. However, I will always remember one of the sayings in this book, "what you think about, you bring about." My thoughts started coming to the surface and I realised I was not paying attention to my thinking over the years. I was constantly getting anxiety attacks, fleeting thoughts, but they would come with an "edge".

It was these thoughts that led me to a healing journey and to be honest if it were not for our two children, I am not sure would I have known about this wonderful healing modality. It was Ava's journey that showed me that it truly works with time, and it was Jack's doing that led me to reach out for help. I could not take anymore.

It all came to a head when I was going to work one morning and getting my two beauties ready. Jack being Jack, laid back, no panic, no rush, was heading to the bathroom and I was telling him to hurry on. It was in that moment, what I now know as a PTSD flashback of the accident occurred. But my mind was telling me that was what I wanted to happen. It could not be further from the truth as it was my biggest fear.

Why was I having these thoughts? Was I evil? What was happening? I was scared, really, really scared.

I went to my local doctor and told him what was happening. I thought he would judge me, lock me up and throw away the key. He told me he was quite sure that I was suffering from anxiety and PTSD, (Post traumatic Stress Disorder). He would have me assessed by a specialist in this field. I went for the assessment and was diagnosed with anxiety and PTSD. I went back to my doctor, and had a chat with him. I thought they all got my diagnosis wrong. I kept thinking, "Who can I talk to? Who can I trust? Who will understand me? How can I stop my mind from this constant racing? Why am I having those intrusive thoughts?"

I discussed the possibility of having 'Bio Energy' treatment over the medication offered. He knew about the modality and recommended this path but reminded me it was an immensely powerful treatment. He explained, "The energy treatment has and will bring up stuff and you will heal from it." To me, that meant nothing, as far as I was concerned, I was going to a therapist and they were going to make me better.

So I started my healing journey.…

I went to a local Bio Energy Therapist and he also confirmed that I had Post Traumatic Stress Disorder and anxiety. Honestly, I still did not believe them. I continued with the treatment, continued to seek information on anxiety, went for counselling and it was then my journey began to unfold.

I had no idea that all the answers lay within. I genuinely thought that any illness was an outside force and it was out of my control. My outlook began to change. I was now beginning to see my life more clearly and why it was the way it was. Why was I suffering mentally? Why was my physical body in pain? I began the search, and I researched the mind, the body, the link between both, our thought patterns, symptoms of anxiety, and so on.

When you look in the dictionary, anxiety is defined as worry. To me, this could not be further from the truth. The pattern of truth behind this, I believe commences as an original concern, it then becomes a worry, then fear and then anxiety. By the time it has reached an anxious state, it is twisted and exaggerated from the original concern or worry.

I had absolutely no idea this is what happens to a person when they overstretch their mind or body. This was the scariest process for me — the thoughts and the feelings attaching to those thoughts. No one and I mean no one had ever explained this to me throughout my lifetime. No one ever explained when a mind becomes too busy that intrusive thoughts set in, no one had ever explained that following a horrific trauma that a person can experience flashbacks as their body is still holding onto the shock.

A person can move on with their life but stress, grief, sadness, loss or hurt that is trapped and unhealed within the mind or body, and eventually manifests as some sort of pain either mentally, emotionally, physically, or spiritually if not dealt with. A memory never leaves the body, but the dreaded feelings attached to the pain lessens as healing sets in, freeing the person to move forward not carrying the weight of the world upon them.

Therefore, I chose Bio Energy Therapy as one of the most used and most useful treatments during my recovery. This treatment allows healing to take place holistically aiding the mental, emotional, spiritual, and physical body to heal. This being the anatomy of each one of us whether we like it, know it, want it, or believe it. I could have medicated, it was prescribed, but for me, it would never have allowed the freedom of my emotions to be. I would have suppressed it all, freezing me inside and out, not facing my truths, not dealing with life, further allowing physical symptoms to manifest, possibly causing illness and disease. I do not proclaim to have all the answers, but my journey has educated me on how to overcome my anxiety and this, in turn, is why I pursued a career working with people in this field.

I was as low as any person could ever imagine. I thought I was a goner. I felt crippled. I was scared recovery would not take place. My symptoms were unfolding day by day, symptoms that I buried. I had no idea what was happening each time I experienced an "attack". I never disclosed to anyone what used to happen to my body and mind, not all the time but at times. These experiences frightened me and came with a huge sense of shame, guilt, and horror. Again, I was totally unaware of what was happening was anxiety or PTSD. I was unaware that doing all the things I wanted to do in life without taking care of myself was going to bring my mind to a very fragile mental state.

I was happy working, and I was happy being productive. I was happy going out meeting my friends. I was happy being a mother. I was happy being a wife. I was happy being a homemaker. I was happy looking after finances. I was happy with my lot except I was not happy with my thinking and the feelings these thoughts were bringing. I had totally ignored myself, my wellbeing, my own presence in this world. I had failed to fuel my own tank leaving me totally empty, exhausted and my mind in absolute chaos.

I would have always tried to remain upbeat about life, not truly showing my emotions as this to me would have been a sign of being weak, inferior, vulnerable, and so on. Now, this shows me that I was totally burying my head in the sand, I was failing to show my true self, part of what makes us whole is that when we are feeling emotions, we need to express them.

An incredibly wise lady once told me, to be true to ourselves it is imperative for our wellbeing that we allow oneself to express the emotions each one of us deals with daily — sad, mad, glad and fear. It is our acknowledgement of those feelings that help in our release, not carrying the heaviness going forward. So, if you feel like a good cry, go ahead, and let it out, crying is your strength, not a weakness.

I had started my journey, and sometimes I feared I had opened a can of worms and could not close the lid. All was being revealed from deep inside, and the Bio Energy treatment had brought me to a place where all my symptoms were being revealed. This in turn allowed me to heal mind and body. Thus educating myself going forward facilitated me to bring awareness to our next generation. We are sponges on this earth, and our children absorb everything we do as we did from our parents. It is important for me as a parent to try and break any ancestral patterns, behaviours, anxiety states, negative thought forms that may have harboured my life and in turn, our childrens.

The energy treatment started to reveal the various anxiety symptoms that I had experienced over the years. All unspoken, all obviously unhealed mostly because of my 'ignorance' to what was wrong with me. I did not know what anxiety was. Yes, I would have described myself as a worrier, but that was it. For me, not knowing what anxiety does or is, was the scariest thing. Media today tells us to look after our mental health. This is wonderful but still not enough. People are still unaware that the symptoms they are experiencing are anxiety-related and you can heal from it or them.

Medication is, in my opinion, compounding the stigma that people experience around mental health. Why are people not educated from a young age about the happenings of one's mind should they find themself caught up in the everyday stresses, trauma, injury, disease, or loss of a loved one? Knowledge is power and if you know a little, it will certainly help a lot.

Whilst symptoms vary from person to person, I feel it is so important that I express and explain to everyone some of the symptoms of anxiety.

- Fear of Losing Control
- Fatigue
- Fear of Knives (Killing someone)
- Heart Palpitations
- Fear of Pillows (using them)
- Tingling through body
- Sexual Confusion
- Nausea
- Headaches
- Night Sweats
- Stomach-ache
- Burning Skin
- IBS
- Yawning
- Not wanting to mix socially
- Muscle Tension/Aches
- Not being able to sleep
- Shaking
- Depression

- Ringing in the ears
- Autonomic arousal of the body
- Intrusive thoughts
- Dizziness/Light-headedness
- Feelings of doom and gloom

The above are just some of the symptoms I experienced on my journey. Not knowing what or why I felt them added more to my anxiety. The fear of them fuelled their power over me, so the cycle ensued.

I just want to share some of my story in the hope that if someone reads this and does not know what is wrong with them or why they are feeling the way they are, that it will help in some way.

No, you are not going mad. Yes, you need to slow down. Yes, you need to take care of yourself. Yes you need to find whatever it is that you feel drawn to, to manage your stress. Some may think, ok, I will go to a therapist, have a session, and see how I get on. Anxiety can be so deep-rooted that 'a session' will not get to the root of the problem. This is something that may take time and there are no quick fixes. We are all looking for the quick fix in our lives and society has provided so much instant gratification that we expect this instantly for our wellbeing.

We are human beings. We will experience the sad, mad, glad and fear in our lives and because we go for therapy, this does not by any means say that you are never going to have a fearful day again. This is not true. Working on yourself can and will help you release the baggage from the past to lighten your load in moving forward. It will also show you the habitual behaviour that possibly once served you is no longer serving a purpose for you on your journey. This is where change is required, and we humans are creatures of habit.

A saying I once came across, stated the biggest sign of insanity is doing the same thing over and over and expecting a different result. We have to change our behaviour, habits, diet and thought patterns. This does not come overnight but believe me, we can all be well in mind and body if we just look within and take care of ourselves.

Bio Energy treatment allows healing to take place and worked for me and for that reason, I decided to train in that area. That was back in 2008 and in 2009, I set up my own practice and have never looked back. I see people on a one-to-one basis most of the time but on occasions, I work with various organisations, schools and hotel groups. I have been asked to facilitate meditations, etc. People come to me all the time and some may think that I am fixing them. This is not the case.

As a therapist, I work with you and aid the release of blocked energies stored within one's energy field. This in turn allows the person's healing to take place, enhancing the balance mentally, physically, emotionally and spiritually. A session usually lasts approximately one hour. It is very non-invasive, not much touch in involved and it could entail sound therapy, positive affirmation, visualisation, and scent.

The science behind energy healing is Quantum Physics. Every illness is, I believe, stored within our energy field. Healing involves going back and somehow, scientifically Bio Energy Treatment can allow this to happen, aiding the person to move forward, freer, more at ease and in better health mind and body.

I do not proclaim that I can heal all, but I will do my absolute best in helping every person who wants to help themselves.

Thank you so much from the bottom of my heart for reading my story. I hope somehow it can and will give each one of you some sort of inspiration and know that there is always light, some may have to dig a little deeper but keep going, never "give up." Yes, you may have to "let go" but that's merely our thinking and our habits over what we try to control. For further information on me and my work, please visit my website on www.bioenergyhealthcare.ie. With much gratitude for this platform.

I have included a detailed testimonial from one of my clients below.

Testimonial

Approximately seven years ago, I found myself in unknown territory. I was around twenty-eight years of age, married for a few years with two young children. I was involved in the construction industry and Ireland had found itself in recessionary times, this having a huge impact on me, my marriage, and our life. I was a worker, an extremely hard worker. I knew nothing else. The kids had different ailments, nothing major thankfully but antibiotics were unable to sort it. My wife took our son for Bio Energy Treatment to Marian and this helped him tremendously.

Time passed and my health began to decline. I was young. I was a provider, this cannot be happening... I had constant pressure, on my head, dizziness all the time. I was treated for vertigo and put on medication; this was not working either. I had started a new job and driving was now becoming an issue. I had convinced myself I had a brain tumour and demanded an MRI scan, thankfully too this returned negative, all was clear. I was not getting answers or solutions. I could always fix everything, but this had taken the better of me.

One night, my wife and I were talking, and she suggested I try a Bio Energy treatment with Marian. I was sceptical, but I agreed to go, I would have gone anywhere to get relief.

I made the appointment and met Marian at her home. I did not feel comfortable at all, I hated the fact that she would place her hands on my head, chest and back area, but I went along with it. In the session, Marian suggested I may have anxiety. I instantly told her I had not, but paid up for the four-day treatment and to be honest, did not feel much of a reprieve after the first session.

The following day, I was unsure as to whether I would attend her clinic again, but because I had paid, I returned. We continued with the treatment. Later my wife asked how I got on? I suggested she let me go for a walk up the farm and I would see. It was in those few moments I began to realise this was the first time in months my head was clearer, so from then on I continued at more ease with the four day treatment. This for me being a turning point in my life. Marian suggested I may need to return for more treatments to work on myself, so I sat with it. I would have very conditioned beliefs as a child, some of those needed addressing, but at that time I was unaware that how I was living my life had a bearing impact on my health and wellbeing.

I returned to Marian over the years and it was in one of those sessions that I realised I was actually suffering with anxiety. It had me emotionally crippled, drained, my head was a mess, but one session where Marian and I talked, I realised the symptoms I was experiencing were anxious ones. From there, I never looked back. This was such a relief to know and once addressed, I was not scared of the symptoms anymore, I could move on with my life more at ease, once I had the answers. It was the fear of me losing control and hurting the people I loved most in this world. When Marian explained that she suffered from this and this is what happens when we do not 'fuel our own tank', I no longer felt alone, I knew it was going to be ok. This is where I believe Bio Energy saved my life.

Bio Energy does not stop life from happening, nor should it. Life does have everyday stresses, challenges, encounters, but I know now that I have the tools and know–how to release my stresses and never let my anxieties return to its peak. I am much better at taking care of myself and in turn, I am much more capable of taking care *of the people I love. If I find my stress levels rising, I know I need a session of Bio Energy, this clears me and helps me continue my journey. I have learned so much in relation to myself over time and the benefits of this treatment have saved me. From a sceptic to now a trainee practitioner.* – **Brendan Murphy**

Thank You For The Gift
by Rose O'Connor

Let me tell you a little bit about myself, how I came to do Bowen Therapy, what it is, how it works, what it treats and how it has benefited people over the years in my practice. I will also discuss what to expect during and after a Bowen session along with the principles I follow.

I have included two testimonials as examples of how Bowen Therapy has helped change peoples lives.

My name is Rose O'Connor. I grew up in the country on a farm just outside the town of Ferbane Co. Offaly. I was one of six children. My mother was the principal of a local national school and my father was a farmer. In February 1990, I commenced my nurse training in London. I spent ten wonderful years there. I now live in Moate, Co. Westmeath with my husband Owen and our three wonderful teenage children. I work in Tullamore General Hospital part-time as a nurse and see clients in my practice in Moate. I have been perfecting the Bowen technique for eight years now.

My journey began in January 2011 while driving home from a twelve hour shift at the hospital about four miles from my house. Something happened suddenly. It was like being hit by a bolt of lightning. As dramatic as that sounds, it is true, and I remember it very clearly. I experienced the worst abdominal pain ever. My whole body was in shock. I thought I was going to die and all I wanted was to get home. I could not even put the key in the door. I could feel that my blood pressure was really low and I was as white as a sheet and clammy. I lay down on the couch and thought that this would pass, that I could continue as usual, but this was not the case. This was the turning point for me and so began the start of my recovery, which took nine months. I questioned a lot during this time. I had no choice other than to slow down and listen. What had happened? Still to this day, it is a mystery. Was I going to recover? At my worst, I could not sit, stand, or lie down without extreme discomfort and I could not walk. The traditional medical route was not for me as much as the doctors tried. The pharmaceutical route was not for me either. I had a heightened sensitivity to medications and for me, their side-effects outweighed the benefits.

Was I going to be able to return to work or what was I going to do? I had worked all my working life as an RGN, and I was only a young woman. It was a turning point in my life and a very frustrating time for me. When I was given a diagnosis following nerve conduction studies, my husband Owen found out that there were three therapists in Europe qualified to deal with my diagnoses and one of whom was in Dublin. I travelled up and down to Dublin for months to get treatment and thankfully, it worked for me.

I started looking at complementary health therapies. The body's' ability to heal itself is most extraordinary. Our body's' have an incredible capacity to heal themselves. When you think of this amazing system, there are 30-40 trillion cells in the human body and every second we are alive, these cells work tirelessly to achieve equilibrium, keeping us at or bringing us back to a natural balance. When we abuse our bodies or become ill, cells can be damaged or destroyed, sometimes in large quantities. However, these cells can heal or replace themselves, all to keep the body functioning at optimal levels. The bodies innate healing mechanism can be reset in many ways. No one size fits all. I believe that if you give your body time, attention, the correct environment, and trust that it will heal itself. It will. This has fascinated me and lead me to study various techniques of energy healing over the years. Some of which are listed here: Chakra Healing, Crystal Healing, Healing meridians, Affirmation, and Meditation. I practise self-healing every day and it has become a way of life now.

My first brief encounter with Bowen in 2003 was when my son was a baby. A lady by the name of Marie Burke demonstrated Bowen on Owen Junior to treat constipation. It took seconds. It did not cause any distress to him; in fact, he was very relaxed afterwards and the result from this one treatment was profound. It amazed me. At the time, I was not able to pursue Bowen with a young family and a busy life. I had been saving for a trip to New York which did not materialise.

In 2011 I had the funds and the time to research this a bit more and the family were not as dependent on me. What happened next was synchronicity at its best. I knew then I was on the right path when I sent an email to the Bowen Association in the UK expressing my interest for the next available course and they told me that there was a course starting in Dublin in September of that year. How lucky was I! It was fate. I had prepared myself to travel to the UK to do the course. And now the course had come to me.

The Bowen Technique exists to improve the wellbeing, health, and quality of life of those it treats.

I want to take this opportunity to pay tribute to my father Josie B. Keenan and my mother-in-law Mary O'Connor who have both been a massive part of my life and of my Bowen journey. They were two of my biggest fans. Sadly, we lost them both in the last nine months. They were always so encouraging, supportive and accepting of the technique and I have no doubt that they had their part in me writing this chapter. They craved Bowen and loved to see me coming. They would tell me if they had a pain or an ache or difficulty breathing, and I would do what I could/knew to help. There are many stories and wonderful memories with them both, but the story I wish to tell you about here today is about my father.

My father had gone through treatment for cancer from September to March 2011/2012 and surgery before this. When I started Bowen Therapy, I was still training, and I visited him. He was in bed, so I decided to treat his feet and he quickly began asking questions. What is it, where are you doing it, and can it treat my hands? (He had never mentioned any pain in his hands before.) So, I treated his hands that day. About two months later I went with him for his check-up with the doctor after his cancer treatment. I wheeled Daddy into the clinic room and when the doctor asked him how he was, all he had to say, lifting both arms in the air, opening and closing his hands, was that he had no pain. I was speechless. I could not believe it. The doctor did not get it, but I did. It may seem unrelated to the majority, but I think my father had peripheral neuropathy of his hands, which is quite common post-chemotherapy and that Bowen Therapy was making a huge difference. I will never forget it. All that he had been through and this was his response. I will be forever grateful that when I could not do anything else for them both, I could always do Bowen and I did, whether it was in person or by distant Bowen.

What is the Bowen Technique?

Ozzie Rentsch describes it so well in our Bowtech manual revised edition 2007.

[The Bowen Technique is a dynamic system of muscle and connective tissue therapy. It was developed by Tom Bowen (1916-1982) in Australia. By using small, gentle movements, it stimulates the body to heal itself often profoundly. The Bowen treatment offers tremendous benefits to clients. It is a holistic, individualised treatment. It restores balance via the autonomic nervous system. The autonomic nervous system controls over 80% of bodily functions and it is very susceptible to external stressors, as most people today live in a constant state of stress. The sympathetic nervous system is working overtime. Healing can only occur when the body is assisted in shifting from fight or flight mode to rest, relaxation, and repair mode. Bowen helps with this transition.]

During a Bowen treatment, clients often quickly drop into deep relaxation or fall asleep. By giving your body this deep permission to relax, it could explain in part, the common observation that Bowen sessions seem to reactivate the recovery process in situations where healing from trauma, sickness or surgery has stalled or reached a plateau.

The Bowen Technique allows the body to heal itself with minimal intervention. I would compare it to a computer – by switching a computer on and off you can reboot it. From my experience and observations over the years, I feel the same is possible with the body.

Bowen Therapy aims to balance your body and resolve your aches and pains. Sometimes there is an immediate relief but more often, the body repairs and resets itself slowly over days and weeks following the Bowen sessions. Bowen therapy is a holistic treatment. It treats the whole body, both mentally and physically. It remains a bit of a mystery as to how the Bowen Technique works, but there are many theories. It has been shown to impact the body in several ways. In addition to rebalancing the autonomic nervous system, Bowtech (which it is sometimes referred to) moves and procedures may reset the body to heal itself by activation through the nervous and endocrine systems, among others.

The Nervous System The gentle Bowen movements will stimulate the body's nervous system receptors. These signals stimulate the body to begin its own healing process by activating the parasympathetic nervous system, which encourages the body to relax and muscle tension to ease. It also promotes digestion and with many clients hearing gurgling noises from the stomach.

Fascia is connective tissue which is found just beneath the skin. There is so much research being done now to learn more about this amazing sensory organ. Some people say it is our largest sensory organ in the body.

It is the matrix that attaches, stabilises, encloses, and separates muscles and other internal organs. It plays a key role in muscle coordination, postural alignment, as well as structural and functional integrity. If your fascia is somehow twisted, tight, or even dehydrated, this can affect your muscles and posture. Bowen therapy works primarily on the superficial fascia helping it untangle and in doing so, frees the muscles which it surrounds. Andrew Taylor, the father of osteopathy, described fascia beautifully when he said, "fascia is the living waters where dwells the soul of living man."

Lymphatic System Gentle Bowen movements activate the draining of the lymphatic system, which can include the detoxification and stimulation of the immune system.

What Can Bowen Therapy Treat?

Bowen Therapy is always aimed at treating the whole body. Very often, the cause of pain is different to where you feel it. As the body adjusts and re-balances, the effects can act on many of the body's systems and not just the muscles. Therefore, positive results can be seen with seemingly unrelated conditions such as IBS (irritable bowel syndrome), chronic fatigue and asthma.

Although we treat the whole body, the list below shows some conditions that do respond favourably to the Bowen Technique. This list is in no way exhaustive. If you have a condition that is not listed, please contact me on www.bowen.ie to see if Bowen Therapy can help you.

- Migraine/Headaches
- Hay Fever/Sinusitis
- Asthma/childhood asthma
- Baby Colic and disease caused by trauma at birth,
- Being born premature, feeding difficulties and sleep disturbance
- Baby and childhood problems
- Fertility issues
- Pre and Post-operatively
- Hormonal imbalance
- TMJ (temporomandibular joint)/ or jaw dysfunction
- Sports injuries
- Anxiety and stress
- Digestive system problems/lBS
- Back Pain/Sciatica

- Neck/Shoulder problems
- Carpal Tunnel Syndrome/RSI (Repetitive Strain Injury)/ tennis elbow
- Fatigue/ME (Myalgic Encephalomyelitis)/Depression
- MS (Multiple Sclerosis)

As Bowen therapy addresses the entire body, it can have a wide range of benefits. This gentle non-invasive method has successfully assisted a wide range of health problems. It has helped in preventing unnecessary surgical procedures. The Bowen Technique has been found to achieve excellent results with a wide range of acute and chronic conditions. Some of the ways people have noticed how Bowen therapy has helped them are they experience:

- A unique sense of relaxation
- Reduces stress
- Balances muscular tension
- Increases the range of joint motion and flexibility
- Improves posture
- Better quality sleep
- Helps with the elimination of toxins
- Improves breathing and absorption of oxygen in the lungs
- Reduces chronic pain
- Often improves psychological symptoms
- Improves energy levels
- Strengthens the immune system
- Enhances the body's own innate healing
- Increased sense of calmness and wellbeing

What happens during a session?

I speak to my client, listen, obtain a history and consent, devise a plan of care, discuss this with my client and I ensure they are comfortable and happy with the above before we proceed.

The Bowen session usually involves a few procedures, each of which consists of several sets of moves. Hands-on treatment usually takes 30-45 minutes.

The treatment starts with the client lying on their tummy on a massage table, then on their back. Sometimes they sit in a chair or whatever is comfortable for the client.

The moves are gentle rolling type movements made with the thumbs and fingers at the level of the superficial fascia just underneath the skin on specific points.

Between each set of moves, the practitioner pauses for as many minutes as are needed for the client's body to begin responding to the movements that have been made.

This rest period is an important part of the treatment as it gives the body time to make the subtle and fine adjustments needed.

The lower back is addressed first, then the upper back and then the shoulders and neck.

As Bowen activates the body to heal itself, it continues to work for 5-10 days following treatment and sometimes even longer. It is usually advised to have a course of Bowen treatments consisting of 4-6 sessions. One week apart for optimum results. I would recommend a maintenance treatment once a month or every two months as a rough guideline.

Instructions Following Your Bowen Session

- In the days immediately following a Bowen treatment, you are advised not to sit for more than 30-minutes at a time. A little gentle exercise is encouraged to keep things moving. Moving helps the body to realign itself. Walking is one of the best forms of exercise.

- Ensure you increase your usual water intake to help the process – the more hydrated the body, the better the benefits.
- Trust the technique and refrain from having any other bodywork for at least one week before and after treatment. Bodywork would include:
  - Physiotherapy
  - Reflexology
  - Acupuncture
  - Chiropractic
  - Magnet Therapy
- Refrain from using hot and cold packs during a Bowen session.
- Continue to take medications prescribed by your doctor.

Each individual response is unique to the Bowen technique. Occasionally clients may experience a strong response to Bowen work within the first few days following treatment. You may experience one of the following symptoms or a combination and this is a natural response: emotional release, tiredness, thirst, hot and cold flushes, headaches or body aches and pains. Just be aware of any changes and let me know at your next visit what you experienced.

Bowen is a complementary therapy that is holistic. It treats the body as a whole. I started off practising and working on friends and family. Most of whom will now come back to me when they have a problem. I have treated people who have a real phobia of doctors, having blood taken, procedures carried out and the whole hospital environment. But they will come to me. It is fear of the unknown which I try to alleviate by answering their questions and explaining procedures.

The Principles I Work By

As a practitioner, I am responsible for keeping myself updated, and transmitting my knowledge and skills into practice to deliver the highest possible standard of care to my clients. My main aim is to promote and maintain health and wellbeing within an environment of open communication, mutual respect, and confidentiality, providing a peaceful, comfortable, and relaxed environment where people can relax and be themselves. Empowering them to help themselves and providing simple tools to help them to do so. I see myself as a channel through which healing can occur. I work intuitively and with intention.

I have included two testimonials here as examples of how Bowen therapy has helped change peoples' lives in their own words:

This is an area of my work that I wish to pursue further in the future. I love working with mothers and babies; it is so rewarding to be able to help both. Most babies use crying to communicate and they will continue to cry or show signs that they are upset until their needs are met.

How Bowen Helped Me Conceive

I was trying for a baby for over seven years; I did all the fertility clinic procedures you can think of and finally did three rounds of IVF .... it was horrendous and a very lonely time but the minute I had my first baby I wanted another which was heartbreaking as I knew I probably had to go through more fertility treatment.

To my surprise, I had gotten pregnant a year later spontaneously but unfortunately had a miscarriage. I had hoped I would get pregnant straight after, but it wasn't so and after meeting Rose on a course, we spoke about Bowen Therapy and I was intrigued. I instantly liked Rose and her calming presence and I thought she would be someone I could work with. So, I asked her if she thought she could help me, and she agreed. Both my husband Gary and I met with Rose and following a discussion with us both, we planned together.

My first session of Bowen Therapy was not at all what I expected. It was an exceptionally light touch and the room was silent. For me initially, it was a strange experience because I work as a massage and reiki therapist where it is all soft music and more hands-on treatment, but by the second treatment, it felt great. Rose said she would balance our bodies first and then synchronise them. And that is exactly what she did. It was that simple. After about six weeks and four sessions, I fell pregnant. I could not believe it. I had a perfect beautiful baby boy. When I think of what I went through with IVF and how stressful it was.

There is absolutely no comparison — the simple, natural, relaxing, gentle, and subtle moves of Bowen Therapy are mind-boggling. When our little boy was only a few weeks old, we brought him over to Rose for his first Bowen treatment and he absolutely loved it. He was so relaxed.

We look forward to a Bowen Treatment with Rose as often as we can, which is not nearly often enough as it is hard to juggle a young family and a busy life. But I would not have it any other way. Each time it surprises us. I love it so much I plan to do the course in the future. I am so thankful for meeting Rose when I did. I would recommend Rose and the Bowen Treatment 100%. - **Lisa, Gary Mc Mahon, and baby Eli**

Rachel was one of my case studies. I had only been practising Bowen about seven months when I started working with Rachel. What attracted me to Rachel was she was the same age as me, yet it shocked me the amount of strong medication she was on and her exceptionally long medical history.

My Experience Of Bowen Treatment

Where do I begin …. My name is Rachel Brennan and I first met Rose at the pain clinic where I was regularly attending. It seemed every time I was there, I was diagnosed with another illness on top of the fibromyalgia, which included lupus and rheumatoid arthritis. On this particular visit, I was getting injections into my knees and was due to get my date for my second liver biopsy. I had at this stage taken to the bed for almost eighteen months with the pain I was in. It was unbearable. My youngest child was just gone two years at that time and a family member moved in to help me with my four children. I was on so much medication that I could not remember them all, so I had them posted on two sheets of A4 paper — front and back. Rose mentioned to me she was training in Bowen treatment and explained a little about it and that she needed to practice, so I said I would be interested — anything was worth a shot at this stage as I was not getting any better, in fact it was the opposite.

So off I went to Rose for several visits and to be honest, I did not think anything was happening, but I continued to go. I started seeing Rose in February and by April I was feeling much better than I had in years. Even the kids were commenting on how I was improving, staying up for longer periods, doing more around the house and even going shopping. I was feeling so good, I decided to try and come off the medication under the supervision of my GP. It took me until the July to wean off all the medication and I found the Valium hard but once I decreased the dosage, I had no problem. My personal life was not the best and in the midst of it all, I separated from my husband and moved back to Clare with my four children and never really thought of how Bowen treatment worked for me – as you can only imagine I had so much going on in my life.

In the December, Rose made contact with me and was very surprised that I had moved to Clare. After chatting to her for a while, I was telling her how much my life had improved and I was off all the medication and only took some very rarely. Rose offered to do distance healing the following evening and this is when the penny dropped for me. As I was lying in bed, I could feel my body tingling and I thought to myself, how come I did not feel this the last time, but how could I feel anything when I had been on so much medication that my body was numb.

It's very safe for me to say that Rose O' Connor saved my life. I went from spending the best part of three years in pain and two of those years were in bed, to moving out of a very unhappy relationship and going back home to Clare. While the first two years were difficult, to say the least, I am now a happy, independent woman who went on to school to do Level 5 and progressed to college where I have now my Level 7 degree and I am continuing onto Level 8. I also plan to do a Masters. I have more energy now at forty-eight than I had before I got the Bowen treatment. I continue to get distance healing from Rose when I need it, which thankfully is not very often as I am in the best of health. I cannot praise Rose enough as she saved my life and started me on my journey to a happier life. I will forever be grateful for that day in Tullamore where I met a true Earth Angel in Rose. I would highly recommend Bowen treatment to each one of you. Go with an open mind and believe in it as it does work, and I am living proof of that. - **Rachel Brennan**

Over the years, I have done several courses in Bowen, learning new and different techniques from some of the most amazing and incredibly talented people in the Bowen circle.

They all have their own unique way of teaching and looking at the body and visualising what the body needs. Bowen is something I practise, and it is also my favourite past time. I love going on these courses because I always learn something new and it gives us Bowen therapists time to meet up and connect and share ideas and experiences with like-minded people. I have met some of my best friends through Bowen. I am passionate about what I do, and I am grateful for having the tools to make a difference in peoples lives. It never ceases to amaze me. I love Bowen because it has the ability to transform people's lives for the better, from something so simple as allowing them to have a restful sleep and to wake up energised, to being part of helping a couple conceive, to changing a stressful situation of having a distressed colicky baby in the home to one of calm and peace. I am incredibly grateful for the support and encouragement I have been given along the way and the friends I have met. Some of the many benefits that I have found with Bowen Therapy are:

- It is a natural, safe, gentle, and effective pain relief.
- It is a relaxing therapy that can have profound results.
- Bowen activates the body to heal itself, within the body's own capacity.
- It can be performed on everyone, including pregnant women, babies and the elderly.
- There are no oils used, just gentle touch.
- It can be performed almost anywhere. i.e. In a clinical setting or outdoors.
- There is no risk of an allergic reaction or drug interaction, as all that is needed is a gentle touch.

I have attended several courses and sat in on many webinars about Bowen therapy. These are just some of the courses I attended. **Mind, Body Bowen which was taught by Margaret Spicer and Anne Schubert**. They both travelled from Australia to Ireland. They taught about the inherent wisdom/intelligence of the body as it indicates links between the physical, emotional, mental, and spiritual aspects of our being — the 'felt sense' related to awareness and its role in the releasing of post-traumatic stress.

Working with babies and children, plus adults with residual associated emotional and behavioural patterns were explored as well as looking at Bowen in relation to meridians blockages and how it can be observed and worked on.

Mother and Baby Bowen in Hammersmith taught by John Wilks and Lina Clarke. John Wilks is a cranial sacral therapist, Bowen therapist, teacher, and author.

John became interested in this area following the birth of his last child. It was a difficult birth and his wife sustained a fractured coccyx from the event. He also spent a few years working with couples in a fertility clinic and assisting couples with fertility issues. He has written several books, including a book dedicated to women, pregnancy, and birth.

Lina was the first-ever doula I meet. A doula is someone who works with a woman before, during and after birth. Lina was deeply passionate about natural/home births and supporting mother and baby throughout ensuring that the experience was a wonderful experience for mother, baby and all the family.

The Sports Injury Course with Robyn Woods during her visit to Ireland from Australia. I found it extraordinary meeting this lady. She was a neighbour and family friend of Tom Bowen and she had many stories to tell. She said of Tom Bowen 'we were astounded by his ability to read the body and know just what little moves on certain muscles could heal all sorts of problems. It did not seem to matter if it were my fathers' elbow, or indeed a horse or a cow!' She remarked that it was wonderful when he worked on her beloved horses. Their attitude and ability always improved after his magic touch.

I have been extremely fortunate to have met and spoken to **Ozzie and Elaine Rentsch**. Ozzie was asked by Tom Bowen on his deathbed to teach his work throughout the world. Tom described Bowen 'as a gift from God'. Ozzie and Elaine have done him justice. An extraordinary couple who have brought Bowen worldwide. It is now being taught in over forty countries. They are both in their eighties and continue to travel and teach the original Bowen Technique or Bow Tech as it is sometimes referred to. There is a documentary dedicated to Tom Bowen and his work in progress which should hopefully be out in the next few years. It is called 'These Two Hands'.

TMJ dysfunction taught by Ron Phelan: Ron looked at the body and how the temporal mandibular joint can be responsible for a wide range of conditions. It is one of the most used joints in the body. It is associated with talking, eating, and swallowing and many, many other functions. How treating this one joint can have a domino effect on the rest of the body.

The Art of Bowen By Alistair Mc Loughlin: Alistair based his 'Art of Bowen' teaching on three elements. Assessment, Correction, and Confirmation. He also introduced us to McLoughlin Scar Tissue Release MSTR.

After this, I became interested in Scar Tissue Release and attended a course with Jan Trewartha, who taught the Sharon Wheeler Scar Tissue Release course. I am privileged to be among the first twelve people to be taught this technique here in Ireland in November 2019. We saw some transformations on this course. This too is a gentle touch therapy with incredible results. Scar tissue therapy works on healed wounds. Regardless of how long ago the accident, injury or surgery happened, there is always healing to be gained.

I have found when you combine working on the matrix of the superficial fascia with gentle touch, extraordinary things happen.

I have always been interested in the power of touch. Touch that is wanted causes the release of oxycontin. It helps to nurture feelings of trust and connectedness and it also reduces cortisol the stress hormone. Twenty seconds of affectionate touch is enough to trigger the release of oxytocin. This kind of touch signifies warmth and intention. Research has shown that it takes eight to ten touches a day to maintain physical and emotional health. Studies show 'that positive touch signals safety and trust, it soothes'. This is from Hey Sigmund aka Karen Young Psychologist www.heysigmund.com.

Another example of the power of touch is presented below.

Kangaroo care (skin-to-skin/mother and baby) was initially utilized as a lifesaving practice for premature infants, but there are over one hundred and sixty research studies on the full-term new-born that document the need and benefits of Kangaroo care. It is promoted as an essential element of new-born care to save and improve all new-born lives by UNICEF, Save the Children and the WHO.

This has overwhelming benefits for both mother and baby. Helping the bonding process, it is also seen as powerful medicine. The mother's heartbeat, rhythm and scent are all comforting to the baby and vice versa. When your baby feels your skin on theirs, their brain releases oxytocin which helps stabilizes their cardiovascular system, reduces stress and makes them feel calmer and safer. It is the perfect environment for the baby to thrive, helping with regulating the baby's temperature, feeding, and sleeping patterns.

Bowen has brought such joy, happiness, and abundance into my life and those of my clients. I treat people instinctively and I know I have been extremely fortunate to have been given this gift, which I appreciate and thank God for every day.

If someone were to ask me how I would describe Bowen in just a few lines, I would say Bowen resets the body, bringing the body into a deep relaxation state where energy can flow to where it is needed to help the body to balance and regenerate itself. That is if you would listen and allow it to do so. The power is in your hands. Just trust the technique.

I feel very excited about what the future has in store for me on this journey.

I hope you have enjoyed reading this chapter and that it has given you an insight into what Bowen Therapy is all about.

If you wish to know more about Bowen Therapy, please contact me Rose O'Connor RGN/Bowen Therapist located in the heart of Ireland.

F/B bowen.ie
email rose@bowen.ie
Website www.bowen.ie

The Universe Held My Hand
by Una McNerney

If anyone would have told me when I was in my early thirties that I would be doing the work that I am doing at present, or that I would have gone down a path of energy work, I would probably have said "absolutely no way" after I pulled myself up off the floor from laughing. It just was not on my agenda and to be honest, I knew nothing and cared little about it. I guess I would have been under the impression that the people who were into that kind of work were a bit 'Airy Fairy', and that certainly was not me, or so I thought.

In 2005 that changed a little for me, at the time I was thirty-eight years old, married with two small children and I was working in a medical factory. I recall this particular weekend when I was visiting my Mum, and sitting at the table just glancing out at the sea through the window, and this thought came strong in my mind, 'Universe, there is something more out there for me.' I knew that I was not fulfilled in my work life, don't get me wrong, I was very grateful for my job and my hours and that I had every weekend off but I just felt a little empty. There was a Galway Advertiser newspaper on the table in front of me and I opened it and glanced through it and came across an advertisement for Reiki Level 1 training which was happening the following weekend. I did not know anything about Reiki but felt that I was drawn to do it so I made contact with the lady and booked my place. I did not tell anyone about this not even my husband. I remember distinctly the morning of the training, pulling up outside the lady's house and this overwhelming fear came over me. What was I doing? I hadn't even told my husband where I was, there could be anyone in this house and I may never be seen again. All these crazy thoughts were coming fast and furious, so I got on my phone and rang my husband and gave him the address where I was and explained what I was doing and that if I had not got back to him in the next five minutes, to come and rescue me, and yes, as you can probably gather, my husband is a very patient, understanding man.

It seems funny now as I recall it as clear as day, and how nervous I felt as I took these steps to her door. A lovely, smiling lady answered the door and I began to breathe again as I let my shoulders drop, and I knew that everything was going to be okay. I did contact my husband to put his mind at ease. We made our introductions and then she said there was supposed to be two more people coming, but they cancelled that morning. A sense of relief came over me as I thought obviously she is not going to run it with just one person and felt quite comfortable to go home to my safe space and say "Ah well it wasn't meant to be". Then my bubble was burst and she said "we might as well start!" and I meekly replied "Okay".

That day I had a huge emotional shift and I still recall the words she said as I sat there in floods of tears. "Now I understand why the other two cancelled". It took me a long time to process what exactly had happened on that day. Although I knew something had shifted in me because of the strong emotions that came to the surface, I was apprehensive of moving forward with Reiki as I did not want other people to experience the tears and strong emotions I did, as a part of me believed at the time that this was a bad thing and that maybe in some way it was best to keep your emotions hidden and suppressed. It was quite a while before I came to the realization that what had happened was actually a huge healing for me. I tell all my Reiki students this story and always welcome them with a big smiling face just in case they have any of the fears that came up for me. It was the beginning of my journey, even though I did not realize it at the time. It was four years later before I experimented with the knowledge that would really set me on a path I knew I would not be able to pull away from as I was well and truly hooked.

In 2009 while still working in the medical factory, a work colleague of mine who also wanted to experience more from life and wanted change, but like me did not know exactly what that was to mean told me about a course she was doing at the weekends. It was a diploma course in Indian Head Massage which was quite an in depth course which also covered anatomy and physiology, professional conduct and business awareness. I could feel her excitement as she spoke about it and I was happy for her that she was doing something which was moving her towards her goals. Then she said, "Una, you would really love this course. Why don't you look into doing it?", and that day, another seed was planted. Even though I knew nothing about it, I felt an excitement that it might be something I would enjoy, but also that I would be learning a new skill and let's face it, who does not love a nice head massage. The next day I looked up the course and signed up for the next enrolment. A part of me was nervous as I knew there would be a lot of book work, especially with the anatomy component but a part of me just needed something to move towards, something that would bring some spark back that I had been yearning for.

The course was indeed interesting. I loved the practical side more than the theory of learning of the bones, etc. but I knew that I had to embrace it all and hope that exams would be passed. I will never forget one particular day when we were having a class and instead of our usual teacher, another lady came in to take the class instead saying that she was covering the class for the day. Little did I know that this lady was going to change the path of my life in a few small hours, just by the wonderful stories she was telling us about her time in India, and how the families in India used head massage from generation to generation, so a grandmother, mother, child would all be sitting on floor, grandmother at back, then daughter, then child and each of them massaging the one in front of them. What a beautiful concept. It was just a way of life for them and not just women but men as well, but what really grabbed my interest was when she started speaking about Chakras, (energy centres in the body) and she went through each of them and spoke about them in great detail, where they were located in the body and what their purpose was.

To say I was like a child at Christmas was an understatement. I was probably sitting there with my mouth open as I soaked in every word she spoke and wished the class would never end. I had never heard anything like this in my life. It was not anything that was ever taught at school — definitely not at any of the classes I attended, and I was smitten. I never had the privilege of meeting this lady again and wondered if she would ever know how much her class impacted my life. I am so grateful to her for really starting me on this journey and also so I am mindful as I now run classes of my own and know first-hand how my words may influence someone else's life the way hers influenced mine. And so, began my journey into the world of energy and like everything that happened prior to this, it was like my life was taken on its own journey, a journey with a sequence of events.

The next leg of my journey was to train in Bio Energy in 2011, and again, how this came about was just a tad strange, to say the least. Since finding out about our energy system, I had read some books to help me get a better understanding of it and this particular day I saw a piece on the front page of the Connacht Tribune about a talk that was happening in the Clayton Hotel Galway by Michael O'Doherty about Bio Energy and family health. I was intrigued but when I looked at the date of the talk, it was dated three months earlier, which I felt had to be a misprint on the paper as it was front page. I could not make sense of it and there was a mobile number of a girl in Galway who was organizing the event, so I rang and said I would like to book into the event. She had no idea what I was talking about, and I explained that it was on the front page of the newspaper and she said that it should not be, that it was supposed to happen three months ago but they had to cancel the event. They obviously had made a mistake by printing it again that week. Anyway we begun a lengthy conversation, and she told me she had trained as a bio energy therapist with Michael and was more than happy to answer any questions I had. She asked me if I would be interested in training and I told her I did not even know what it was and that I was not that type of person. I believed that people who worked in this field had a special calling and I definitely did not have it. She felt that the fact that I made contact with her showed I had some interest and she gave me the email address of the organisers to get in touch with, which I did.

One of my first questions was whether this is something you are born with or could anyone become a bio energy therapist? I definitely did not feel like I was born with any special gift but if it was something I could learn, I would be eager to learn as much about it as I could. Needless to say, I began my training and looked forward to the many weekends heading off to Clare to this fascinating course. I learned a huge amount as we covered some Qigong and learned a lot about our breath and diaphragmatic breathing, our organs and connecting more with our body, and of course, the practice sessions would be amazing.

I remember one particular practice session and Michael our teacher would choose different students each time to work on and this time it was my turn. He was showing us the protocol on the legs and feet. As I sat there with Michal working on me, I could feel this coldness coming down from my hip area on my left side and working its way down my legs to my feet. It was the strangest thing and the first time I felt what it was like to feel energy moving through my body. As this was happening, he said I had an old injury in my lower back, hip area, which I could not pinpoint at that particular moment, but knew that something was releasing from there as he was working on me. It wasn't until after the weekend that I linked it to an accident I had a few years previous, but obviously there was some stuck energy there that had released that day. I find this intriguing as I work with people and feel things around parts of their body like their ankles or shoulders and they have old injuries that the energy seems to have remained stuck there.

I remember one particular time I was doing a treatment on my husband and he had been in a serious accident six months previous where he had a broken collarbone and fractured ribs. I was clearing down his arm from his shoulder, he could feel something shifting from his collarbone area and moving out the hand and I could feel this heaviness there also. I worked on that area until I felt it clear. We must remember that the body goes into shock when a traumatic accident happens and although his collarbone had knitted back completely, there was obviously old stuck energy there that needed to be released. I think what I love most about energy work is that it is never dull or boring. Every person that I have had the pleasure to work with, brings with them their own unique energy.

A big part of my work is staying present with each individual as they talk about what is going on for them in the moment and for me I feel that what is happening often in the present moment is a repercussion of something that happened many years previous, even going back to childhood. For many people, this can be hard to make sense of. I remember having a particular client one time who came to me for Bio Energy. Every treatment begins with discussing what is going on or the symptoms that are showing up. This gentleman was having hospital treatment for kidney issues for over a year. As I spoke to him, I mentioned that our kidneys hold our fears and often this can go back to childhood. With that, he opened up about his childhood and how both his parents drank heavily when he was a child. Whenever they did, there would always be a huge row before the end of the night and how he was very fearful as a child as he was always on high alert since he never knew when things were going to explode in the family. He said he still gets phone calls occasionally to collect them from somewhere as the drinking still continues. He would never have related any of his issues to anything from his past and found it hard to believe that what happened as a child could affect him now. The more I spoke to him about the mind-body connection, the more he could relate and make sense of it. This really gave him the power to be able to stand up and look after himself now as an adult and maybe speak to his parents about how he felt. He was still reliving his younger days every time he got a phone call to pick them up and he was feeling the same fear in his body as he did back then. He acknowledged its affects on his body.

In 2013, I met one of the guys I trained with in Bio Energy and he was telling me he was completing his training in The Hidden Mind which is looking more into the subconscious mind. He was looking for case studies to work on for his exams. Myself and my two children became his case studies. I was intrigued with it all and what came up for each of us in the sessions. Needless to say, my curiosity for learning more about this work led me to make contact with the lady who was organising the training.

This course was taught by Tom Griffin and Silvia Henrich, and when we were doing our Bio Energy training, Tom came in one day and gave us a talk about the hidden mind which was fascinating, but he was not teaching it at that time. Tom Griffin and Michael O'Doherty were the two people who brought Bio Energy to Ireland. Tom continued on his work in learning about the Dawson programme and went on to create The Hidden Mind Investigative and Corrective Sound Program. I completed my training in 2014. It really did open up my mind to so much. It made me realize how powerful our subconscious is.

We mistakenly think our conscious mind is running the show but how wrong we are. Our subconscious mind holds every memory and experience we have ever had, good and bad. It is also where our beliefs about life are stored and the more I continue to do this work, the more I realize how big a part our belief system plays in our life without us even realizing it.

To say I loved learning about anything related to energy work and the mind-body connection is an understatement. Apart from the time I spent with my kids, I was at my happiest when I was getting into my car heading off on an evening or a day course to learn something new in this field and the loveliest part was spending time with like-minded people. It can be lonely sometimes when you are doing this work and don't feel you have anyone to chat with as the things I was learning about were not mainstream conversation and I was very careful about who I could open up to.

I also loved reading books to gain more knowledge in this field and one of the books I loved was Louise Hay's *You Can Heal Your Life*. In 2016, I did a two day Heal Your Life workshop with Eileen Claire in Co. Clare. There were six of us doing the workshop. I was feeling both excited and nervous as I had no idea what to expect. Eileen made us all feel very comfortable and throughout the day, we all got to get to know each other through various exercises we were doing. It's amazing how you can let all your barriers down when you feel held in a safe space, which we all did; each of us shared our thoughts and feelings on things that had really impacted our lives in one way or another. Some things had never been shared before, as everyone has their own story that they may not feel too comfortable sharing and we hold on to it in our body, but here it was different. There was no fear of being judged or criticized. It was just about allowing us all to open up to allow healing to happen. I just knew by the second day that I wanted to train in this work to be able to facilitate and teach the philosophies of Louise Hay.

Now to put this into a little perspective for anyone who has never met me, even people who know me; for me to say that I wanted to teach anyone anything was both laughable and cryable for me. Even as I said to Eileen that I was interested in doing the course, I could hardly put the words together. I was a quiet person and had a huge fear of speaking in front of people. In a one-to-one situation I could manage but if I was in a group setting, I would feel physically sick and tearful if I knew I had to speak. All I could think of was that this is a huge investment to make if I couldn't deliver workshops at the end of it, but deep in my heart I knew that this would be life-changing for me and I wasn't wrong. Something changed for me at that two-day workshop. I had not realized it at the time until I was driving home in the evening and about ten minutes into the drive, with no radio on, I just started belting out the chorus of *Bright Eyes* by Art Garfunkel

Bright eyes, burning like fire
Bright eyes, how can you close and fail?
How can the light that burned so brightly?

Suddenly burn so pale.
Bright eyes

And I didn't stop belting it out until I pulled up in my driveway an hour and a half later. Please understand that this is not a normal thing for me and that particular song would not have been a song that I had heard in many years and was by no means a favourite of mine. I am by no means a singer but I have to say, it felt quite liberating. That day at that course, my throat chakra opened and for people who may not know anything about chakras, it is an energy centre located at your throat and when it's open, you have the ability to speak openly, communicate easily, be able to speak your truth and for me and many, many other people my throat chakra was blocked all my life. I do believe that is very much an Irish thing, to be seen and not heard, or be afraid to voice an opinion for fear of being mocked or laughed at.

Again this comes back to beliefs that are formed when we are younger. It's not that anyone ever said to me to that my opinion was not valid, it's just a belief that I held all my life and after feeling safe enough to express myself at the course, it allowed me to unblock old energy there. A few months later, I was driving down to the beautiful Spanish Point, in County Clare to begin my training as a Louise Hay workshop facilitator. As I stood out of my car on a beautiful May day, looking out at the ocean and smelling the sea air, I vowed that I was going to get as much out of this course that I possibly could and as I stared at the high waves beating against the rocks, I felt that this ocean was going to take my mental garbage far out to sea. I was well and truly ready to let go of long-held beliefs that had not been serving me.

As I look back now on that week in Spanish Point, I can't help but feel blessed to have had such a wonderful opportunity. I think there were about nineteen of us who did the course, from Ireland

and other countries and the bond that was formed between us all was amazing. We all supported each other in our fears, tears and laughter. Each of us left at the end of that week as different people to the people who walked in there that very first day. Once you become aware and are willing to let go of limiting thoughts and beliefs that may be holding you back, magic happens.

There were so many highlights of that week but the one that really made me realize how powerful this work is, was when towards the end of the week, Eileen gathered us to tell us that the following day we were all going to give a forty-five minute presentation of one of the parts of the workshop. We got to choose which part and how we wanted to present it. We would be grouped into groups of four and each one delivering their presentation to their particular group with Eileen looking on. Under normal circumstances, this would have been all my worst nightmares coming true — having to present anything in front of anyone but I was actually looking forward to it and was super excited to head to my room to prepare for it. The following day I presented my workshop on the 'Inner child', and it just felt natural to me. I know this may sound strange for someone who was afraid to speak, but this is what changed for me, and I honestly feel that if someone like me could make this wonderful change in my life that there is indeed hope for everyone.

I have run many workshops on Louise Hays philosophies since then and I have seen amazing changes in people who have attended. It's very easy to be passionate about something that you know has helped you and in turn, can help others. I feel that without a shadow of a doubt, I would probably never have been comfortable to put myself into a situation where I would be speaking to groups of any age, so it would be fair to say that both me and my work have flourished since doing this course. It began to open up other avenues that had never been on my radar, like working with children. I guess that's where my journey of meditation and mindfulness began. In hindsight it probably began much before this as I always enjoyed time in quiet reflection and always felt that it was not always important to speak just for the sake of speaking, but I was a great listener and often heard things people never had to say.

I think especially after my training in Louise Hay, I kept thinking, my God imagine if kids were taught this in school, if they were taught that it was absolutely okay to totally love yourself, every part. Because it is in those primary years that kids begin to form these beliefs about themselves — they are not good enough, not smart enough, not good looking enough, not thin enough and the list goes on….. That is what ignited in me this passion for letting them know, which started with my training as a Connected Kids Tudor which was very much about teaching kids meditation and many skills to help children self-regulate.

I really felt that it was so important to instil more positive beliefs in children as it is between the age of five and twelve that kids begin to form beliefs about themselves. Some studies show that it is even younger and I knew first hand how negative beliefs about ourselves can absolutely affect our lives in so many ways which made me quite passionate about sharing my knowledge with children. I was lucky to have had many opportunities to work with children in a school setting and run mindfulness and meditation camps during school holidays with my main emphasis being to connect children more with nature as I feel this is so important.

I was also privileged to have met Louise Shanagher who was teaching creative mindfulness classes for children. After chatting with her, I decided to train with her. Her work really resonated with me about being able to bring more kindness and compassion into mindfulness practice with children and adults.

46

In 2017, I trained to become a master practitioner in Positive Energy Tapping which is a method to improve the flow of energy through the energy body by gently tapping different points in our energy system, also known as meridians. Working with positive set up statements we ask, "what do you need right now to make you feel better?" It's a great way of dealing with fears and worries by asking yourself, "What energies would help you deal with that problem that resonates with you?" Positive or modern energy tapping is a wonderful way for making an enormous difference to a child's life. It's easy to learn, and children are very in tune with their energy states, much more than adults and they have a wonderful imagination. I would invite the children to see what they feel they need to empower themselves, so it could be words like confidence, patience, safety, fun.

I worked in one school for a few years and was lucky enough to have the same students for quite a while and really got to know them on such a deep level. As a group we shared laughter, tears and worries. As a part of every class, I would get the kids to choose a positive affirmation card out of the deck which has a lot of cards in it and I would explain to the children that we often pick the card that we need at that time. I had one particular boy who was quite excitable, who often found it difficult to settle in the class and whom I was especially fond of, but nearly every time he picked the same card, "I AM CALM", and every time he would say to me, "Can I pick another one? I don't want this card." I would say "No, this is the card your energy chose today and what you need." It almost became a standing joke in the class as each child picked their own, but what I found was really amazing and made my heart melt was when in one of the classes I asked the kids to make their own affirmation card of what they felt they needed the most and design it in whatever way that they wanted. The boy I had mentioned showed me his card. I nearly fell off my chair, he had created a beautiful affirmation card of his own, "I AM CALM," as deep down he knew this is what he needed. Needless to say, we all shared a little laugh and I felt so proud that he was so in tune that he knew this. We also shared so many amazing meditations led by the children and to say they were AWESOME is an understatement. They have such imagination and were so creative in bringing us on journeys that I personally will always be grateful for and feel blessed to have had such experiences.

On one particular day, I was working in Limerick with a group of kids and we were doing some positive energy tapping. One of the girls in the group said she had done something similar before with another lady. She explained to us what it was about, which of course aroused an interest in me. When I got home later that evening I looked up the treatment and the name of a lady in Limerick who was trained in it. Patricia Insley was that lady. I made contact with her and we had the most amazing conversation. I related so much to what she spoke about and she told me about how she had started off on her journey. She spoke about Accunect® which really resonated with me. It felt like a huge amount of individual therapies accumulated under one umbrella and I was curious to find out more.

Accunect®

Accunect® was founded by **Dr. Don Ka'imi Pilipovich, DAc, LMT and Sarah Simonis** and is a licensed trademark of Future Medicine Today. The extract below was taken from my Accunect training manual.

[Accunect® means: **Acc** comes from Chinese Medicine Wisdom (and other ancient systems), **U** for 'you', and **nect** for connection to your client, to universal consciousness, and to the power of transformational healing and alchemy or change. Accunect® is a complete energy healing system based on the principles of ancient acupuncture theory, quantum physics, as well as the essential connections between body, mind, spirit, and universal consciousness. The functioning of our body is affected by stress of all kinds. When stress from accidents, injuries, emotional trauma, and toxins affect the nervous system and the biochemistry of the body, correct functioning is compromised, and disease follows. Accunect® is a way to find the keys to unlock your healing ability and to address areas of stress, whether physical, mental, or spiritual. This allows the nervous system and biochemistry of the body to resume normal function so healing can take place.

The first principle of Accunect® is that our perception of reality is a product of our unique experiences and our beliefs and expectations about the world. Since we all have different histories, we all have different experiences of reality. Our individual experiences cannot be a true reality if everyone has a different experience.

The second principle of Accunect® is that our beliefs about the world affect our physiology. If we change our perceptions and change our beliefs, our physiology responds.

The third principle of Accunect® is that our minds are connected to universal consciousness, that we are all one with infinite potential and God consciousness. Our mind/energy fields interact with the zero-point field that connects everything to the universe.]

As an Accunect® practitioner, I observe the potential for more balanced energy and physiology using intuition and/or muscle checking. I then hold this observation as a mental focus or suggestion to the body–mind that it could function in a more balanced way. This suggestion is imprinted into the person's body-mind by using gentle tapping over the head and heart. Tapping over the head stimulates the brain and the nervous system, and tapping over the heart stimulates the heart energy field and the acupuncture meridian system. Body, mind, and spirit are all connected. The nervous system controls the body, but our mind and thoughts control the nervous system.

This is something I feel is so important to realize because many people, including myself, go through stressful times. This stress can result in our mind taking us on a journey of fear and worry, which can cause havoc with our nervous system, which in turn, affects our physical body. We all have our own unique health map as we all have our own unique experiences of life and I guess, what I loved and what enticed me to do this training is that it really looks at so many different aspects of what is ready to shift energetically for the person. I have personally found through working with Accunect® that our beliefs can really hold us back. I would have known this from previous work that I have done. Still, it has really shown up quite strongly in this work. Some beliefs are so strongly engrained in us from our childhood as they have been passed on from generation to generation and can be difficult to shift.

I have just added a few testimonials from some people I have worked with.

Testimonial

My daughter and I were both treated with Accunect® and it is hard to put into words how we felt after the treatment. My daughter was going through a tough time at school and since having three treatments, has appeared more open-minded, lighter, and happier. Una explained very well 'what was coming up' for her during her sessions and explained how she might look at things differently. She explained it so well in a child-friendly way. For me, it brought deep feelings 'to the surface' to be met and released. I personally could not believe how my body reacted by releasing congestion from my system. The feelings that I was finding hard to digest were being released and I felt so much lighter and more aware of how much I was holding, which was not good for me. Una was amazing and so compassionate and reactive to the emotions that were coming up during the session. I would highly recommend Accunect®.

Testimonial

I took my daughter, who was three years old to see Una as she had been suffering from severe constipation and stomach cramps. She was hysterical with pain when we were going to see Una. When we arrived, Una was so warm and welcoming, and I was a very emotionally exhausted Mom which Una picked up on. Una began working on my daughter asking me questions about her and she calmed and gained relief at the session. She left Una so much happier and lighter than when she arrived. She slept that evening after the treatment, and I could see it was from her treatment as this was not her normal routine. She was so much more relaxed and calmer. Una continued working with her both in person and from a distance. I would always know after Una did a distant healing. Stillness would come upon her, often drifting into a calm sleep. I could see how peaceful the sessions were making her and I had some sessions too after speaking with Una. I could understand how important it was for me as her Mum to be in a better space also, as if I am stressed out, my daughter is going to feed into the energy of that. Una and Accunect® made a huge contribution to my daughter as she never screamed or writhed in pain after Una worked on her. Una helped us both so much, and for this I am profoundly grateful.

Testimonial

I had a distant Accunect® session with Una, which I found extremely helpful. I must admit I had my doubts about distant healing before my session. I felt very relaxed during the session and felt heat in certain areas — which afterwards when we spoke, I found out these were areas she worked on (amazing). When Una spoke to me afterwards, her explanation of what she worked on for me was excellent and really resonated with me, particularly in what was going on in my life at the time. I look forward to working with Una again and would recommend Accunect.®

I also continued with my Reiki training and became a Reiki Master in 2018 and had the privilege of training and attuning many students to Reiki Level 1 and Reiki Level 2. I look forward to this so much as it is just so great to see people so passionate about learning techniques to enhance their own wellbeing and the wellbeing of their family. Sometimes I pinch myself at how far I have come on my journey since my first introduction to Reiki. Like I said earlier, this was nothing I ever foresaw me doing, it just seemed to unfold in front of me like a rug — knowing that once it began to roll, there was no stopping it. I won't say there have not been kinks in the rug along the way, but again, that was very much a part of my journey, getting me to go to a deeper level of understanding.

I have been privileged to work with so many amazing people most of whom I haven't named, but you know who you are and I will be always be privileged and grateful for the part you have played and continue to play in my life.

I truly hope that something in this chapter resonates with you. For me, I am so grateful to have been given this opportunity to share some of the amazing therapies that have impacted so much on my life and really helped me along my journey of wellness. My name is Una Mc Nerney. My business is Anois Holistic Therapies. Anois is the Irish word for 'Now' which is what I encourage— for people to become more present in their life.

https://www.Facebook.com/Anoisholistictherapies/

My Other World
by Marie Cronnelly

Rural west of Ireland 1984, I was a young girl of eight years of age. I had a feeling of something but not knowing what it was. I was half afraid of it, half curious by it. I sometimes thought and felt I was strange, different from the rest of my siblings — three older brothers and three younger sisters. I felt at times I was not a typical eight year old, or was I? I could pick up on other people's energy and wondered did everyone feel like this? I also wondered what could I do about it and why me?

I was a bit of a worrier. I do not know how I got it, but I did. I worried mostly about other people, never me. I worried when my parents would go for a walk in the evenings together — would something happen to them when they were out? What if they got hit by a car? I would ask them what time they would be back. God love them, they both worked so hard, they just wanted a half an hour to walk and chat. If they were not home when they said they would be, I would be waiting at the gate for them, relieved when I could see them coming up the road. Then I was fine again, and go back to being a happy little kid, just like the rest of my family, until it would happen again, this was the pattern of my early childhood.

I remember being in first class and there was talk about the world coming to an end. We were brought to the church by our teacher, a lovely nun, I must add. She had us praying decades of the rosary to save us. I would then go home and lie awake for hours wondering if the world was going to end tonight! Now, I had a very normal, happy, upbringing, but I had a predisposition for anxiety and praying in a church to save us did not help!

Looking back on it now from an adult's view, I was connected to something higher and I was sensitive to it. I began questioning everything around me. I thought it was possible that our reality was in fact a figment of someone else's, maybe God's imagination. My son, Riley, asked the very same question to his dad one day. His dad replied "It is entirely possible. Renee Descartes, French Philosopher put forward the argument that 'I think, therefore I am'. so it might be hard to have our own imagination if we were the figment of someone else's." Descartes found that he could not doubt himself that he himself existed, as he was the one doing the doubting in the first place.

On the other hand, I still wanted to know why the days of the week were called the days of the week, why was the sky blue, why do we exist, what does heaven look like — all the questions an eight-year-old would ask. But bearing in mind, we did not have internet but more being told to go into the sitting room and look up the children's Encyclopaedia. After spending hours and hours trying to look up all the answers for all the random questions in my head and not finding some of them, I would ask my mother and she would tell me to run off outside in the fresh air, like so many other busy Irish mothers, taking care of nine of us, and at times our two grandmothers and a granduncle. There was a lot of love and respect for our elders and it was something I loved to watch, listening to them and their stories and how life was difficult back then. I saw strength in them, and I took their strengths.

From a young age, I found a technique for myself that would help me sit with my many thoughts and feelings. My brother had a pigeon coop at the back of our garden where he would let pigeons go and retrieve them again back into their coops. I loved to watch this; my first love of nature. I would sit up on the tin roof of the coop. On a sunny eve, it was even more special. The tin on the roof would heat up and I would climb up the back of it and would just sit there gazing out into the fields and up into the moving clouds passing by. One of my favourite quotes I tell my young students is that *Our thoughts are like clouds, they are only passing by. (Louise Shanagher, Mindfulness & creative arts lecturer).*

I could completely self-regulate myself in the form of breathwork. When you breathe slowly and deeply, you start to calm and sit with your emotions. This had a profound effect on me. I was completely calm, relaxed, and content within myself. After that, I loved to go out and explore nature. I would meet my cousin Mary up on the hills and we would walk the hills, talk about everything and spend hours just exploring, coming up with ideas how to make our own perfume, what we wanted to be when we were older and all the lovely things children get to do. We had freedom in nature. We knew we were lucky as some children did not get to experience nature as liberally as we did as kids. We had no mobile phones, we knew when we were hungry, and we knew someone's mother would feed us. I loved that sense of freedom; it was where I felt connected. I loved the smell of the trees after it rained, the smell of ferns as we crossed over hills. We saw rabbits, hares, new-born lambs, collected flowers, made daisy chains, collected ladybirds. We were free!

But as I started to get older, I lost my self-regulation. I stopped practising my mindful breathing. I did not know anyone who knew what it was. I did not know what it was, I just knew I liked it, but I kept it to myself. I was growing up now and I drifted from it. I eventually lost it and my life was different without it. The seeds of anxiety were growing slowly.

I had no one to reinforce it for me, to encourage it, to embrace and to know that it was ok. I was now becoming a pre-teen and wanted to be like everyone else. It reminds me of the TV series Derry Girls, where one of the girls wants to be an individual but does not want to be it on her own. I was that Derry Gir,l "Well I'm not an individual on me own". Thankfully, I did find it again in my adult life and when I did, I did not let it go. I held it, studied, read, meditated, slept with the books. This is where my passion lies — teaching children the tools for life, just like I had, but because it was just me with my thoughts, the skills had faded for me with time.

Without it, I became a bit boisterous (a word to describe someone spirited and at times slightly out of control–like someone with a spring in their step and a song in their heart singing to strangers on the street). I had a lot of energy and needed to do something with it. I wanted to be a risk-taker, a deep thinker, I did not conform and at times challenged myself, including my parents. So off I went to take on a whole new challenge… I joined Monivea Boxing club to my brother's dismay!

I was the only girl in the country to box at that time. I was always the underdog. Some people did not like it. They said it was wrong, what if I got hurt, that girls cannot box, but my father had such a strong belief system. He believed girls have just as much strength, both mentally and physically, so why not. He asked me if I wanted to go back after the first night and I said "YES!" I needed this. I literally could not get enough of it.

While some of the boys in the club would not even look at me, or would snigger at me when I trained, I took that negative energy in, flipped it on its backside and let it out physically in the ring. Sometimes I did not even know where it came from; it was not anger, but more frustration that I could not do the one thing I wanted to do which was to meditate, ironic and contradicting as it sounds. I had an absolutely fantastic coach by the name of Gerry 'Gus' Farrell who had such a belief in me. He would train me just like the boys, no exceptions. When we were there as kids, we were all the same and I respected him for that. Gus and my father were always in my corner, always encouraging me, always showing up for me.

Then the day came, and I had my first tournament, against a boy who was older and heavier than me and oh boy was I tested mentally and physically that evening. 3 x 1.30 minute rounds. I was bricking it. None of the boys in my club were encouraging except for one or two, but Gus and Pops were. I was sitting in my corner looking over at this young lad who was sniggering at me. My heart was pumping out of my chest; my pulse had gone wild. I was wild. I knew I needed to calm down, so I started breathing. Slowly breathing in through the nose, holding it, then breathing out on the exhalation through my mouth. I found it so hard as my heart was literally beating out of my chest. I stayed with it and I kept it up and soon found I acknowledged the feeling which was nerves/excitement/adrenaline/determination. I breathed into it (accepting it) and then released it.

Then the mantras followed in my head, "Everything is going to be ok. Marie, I believe in you, you can do this." I relate to this as my inner child, this little force inside me would come out to me and say its ok, and I believed her, I would look at Pops and Gus for reassurance and off I went to fight (illegally).

I cannot remember very much of the first round except getting hit so hard that my two pigtails wrapped themselves around the whole of my head. I went back into my corner and my head was reeling so much that I wanted to cry, in fact tears started to roll down my cheeks. It was my emotions trying to break out. I was always a bit dramatic anyway. It was the adventurous side to me even at that age. Gus and Pops looked me in the eye and said said,

"You are strong, Marie. You are lighter on your feet than him. He will tire. That was the best of him in those two rounds. Now, go out there and show him what you have!"I swear at times I felt I was part of Rocky movie, or at least wanted to be!

Again, I turned to my breath to calm myself (again). It calmed my deeply emotional mind and it worked. I tired my opponent and managed to get in a few uppercuts and then I heard the bell go. I was relieved I was still standing.

That evening my opponent shook my hand and I felt respect from him. I was pushed out of my comfort zone and I loved it. We drew that night and I went home to show my mother my first ever trophy trophy at ten years of age in 1986. But sadly, boxing came to an end for me. I was now almost thirteen-years-old, and there were no girls to box. I was growing into a teen and it was not safe for me to continue boxing. I knew that and it frustrated me even more. This is where I pay homage to the first female gold Olympian hero Katie Taylor. Her triumph was historical. The pride and respect I have for Katie is even hard to explain. She changed the world for women that day.

I missed boxing, and I missed the training and competitiveness. We always had a punchbag at home and to this day, I have pads and gloves that I take out now and again. Gus is still coaching in Monivea Boxing Club and now trains my son Riley!

Then came the teenage years and as I grew into my teens, I spent many days and night daydreaming, searching for the meaning of life. I had attended an all-girls primary school, and now there were boys. It was confusing for me. I was used to boxing them and putting up my exterior front, always proving myself to them, that I was just as strong as they were. As like many teenagers, it was turbulent at times, and other times were fantastic. I was not entirely unhappy as such and had a great childhood, but I felt a little ungrateful, confused, alone and quite tired at times. I missed the boxing, something to put my energy into.

I found earlier in my teens that I drifted in and out of friends, having not any one set of friends, but still friends with everyone. At times I was very much a closed book. I never opened, I guess I was a moody, tortured teen who no one would understand anyway. But there was one woman I loved to spend time with, that was my granny.

Granny C was very influential in my life. I was drawn to strong people and she was one of them. She was ahead of her time in some respects, and she loved fashion. She would take great pride in her appearance and walked everywhere in her pinafore dress and bright blue Adidas runners! She always had people call to her for chats and as a teen, I would sit and listen to her talk about growing up during the 1916 rising, getting arrested at age eight by the Black and Tans and interrogated for hours thinking she may have been smuggling arms. I sometimes thought had she been given opportunities like we have today, she would have made a fantastic history teacher. So, for me, my journey into mindfulness is also for my ancestry and for all the strong women in my family gone before me.

The later part years of my teens became a little rebellious at times, falling into the wrong crowds and trying to fit in. But I was very fortunate, I still had my friends from national school and we formed solid friendships in my later teens and I am lucky to say these girls are my tribe, they are my best friends and without them, I would be a very different person. We have always been there for each other, through good times and bad. They are the most wonderful friends a girl could have.

I spent a lot of my twenties travelling. Caroline and I went off to Australia age twenty-one and we had an absolute blast. We got a taste for freedom and we experienced so many new cultures, made lots of friends and made the best of our time there. I felt free. I felt good in the sunshine. I had confidence and as if I had no worries. It was like Party Marie was there for on a year long holiday. We were lucky to come home unscathed as we were so naïve at times. I know I burnt the candle at both ends. We had a hectic social life, partying, discos, travelling, drinking. When we would hit a big night out, I would be the life and soul of the night, but the next day would be torturous for me. I always wondered how everyone else would be a bit groggy, but they would shake it off. I, on the other hand, would struggle. It was like my mind could not keep up with my body. The only thing that would help deal with the anxiety is if I went for a swim in the sea. I would use it as a therapy. I could self-regulate again, calm my racing mind and all would be ok until I went and did it all over again the next weekend!

I moved back home to Athenry at age twenty-eight and tried to grow up; I bought a house. It was terrifying but also somewhere for me to put down roots, but at times I felt trapped. It meant I could not get up and leave whenever I wanted. I guess I could but getting a whopper of a mortgage made me think about it a second time. Today, I am incredibly grateful for my home.

I met a wonderful guy named Fergal and not long after we moved into the house, which was then to become our home. Those years of the late twenties and early thirties was great. Fergal was/is a talented musician. We always had fun nights out and lots of parties to go to. We travelled together back to Australia and Malaysia along the way, life was great. We got engaged the day before my thirtieth birthday in 2006. Fergal had surprised me with a beautiful engagement ring he picked himself. I felt blessed. I thought that if I grew up and settled down, all my worries would leave me. We were married in 2007 in Cyprus. We had all our family and close friends with us, and we all had a wonderful time.

I was at times afraid of having children, as I was afraid I could not take care of a child and what if I didn't feel any maternal love towards a child of my own, what if something happened them, how would I cope? No, I was better off not to have children and we carried on going out, travelling, going to parties. Then I began to feel like there was more to my life and maybe having a child would be wonderful. I used to mind my niece and nephew from time to time and I loved having them stay with me. I loved tucking them into bed, reading stories to them, bringing them on day trips, buying clothes for them. I could not have loved them anymore if they were my own. Fergal was great with them, putting on puppet shows and having them laugh themselves silly. It was then when I saw how much love I had for them and all my other nephews that I thought I could do this. We can be parents. Look at our sets of parents, four of the kindest, hardworking, family orientated people you could ever meet.

In 2011, our beautiful baby boy came into our world, a bright shining light called Riley. He is my son and my angel. He has taught me everything about what is important in life. This was a time in my life when I was genuinely happy. But then thoughts would creep in and I felt like someone was going to pull the rug from under my feet. Those thoughts needed to stop from taking over my happiness and self-sabotaging. It was not until I became a mother that I knew I needed to work on myself and understand the real beauty in life. For what we have right now is true happiness and this comes from within. If you are not happy with what you have right now, at this moment in time, you will never be happy, as you will keep tripping yourself up. I know this. I learnt it the hard way! I was living in fear.

I remember taking Riley and my mother to visit my aunt and uncle when Riley was small. I did not have much sleep the night before and when I did try to sleep, my mind was racing and could not switch off. I was in 'flight mode' all that day. We had a lovely visit with my mother's family. I remember feeling extremely hot throughout the day and made excuses for myself to go into the bathroom. I looked at my reflection. I was pale, bags under my eyes and I was sweating profusely. As I looked at myself, I thought "Oh my god, what is wrong with me" I thought maybe I might be having a heart attack. I knew that if I could just get myself home, I would be ok, somehow. I could not eat. I was pushing food around on my plate. All I could do was drink some water. I had a funny metal taste in my mouth. I somehow managed to get through it. When we got in the car, I said to my mother "Please do not ask me what is wrong with me, but I am not feeling well. Will you ring Pops and tell him to meet me at the back door and get Fergal, my brother to take Riley? I need to go into the sitting room." My mother knew straight away something was wrong, but she did everything I asked her to do without question.

We got home to my parent's house, Fergal took Riley. I knew then I could let it out. Once I knew I was safe and in a safe place, I started to hyperventilate; then I started shaking. My heart was again beating out of my chest and the only one I was fighting this time was myself. Both my parents came into the room, they sat either side of me and took my hand into their hands and rubbed my back and told me to breathe. Once all the adrenaline left my body, I was calm, but shattered. I remember just breaking down crying to them, asking them why this happens to me. I was like that eight-year-old girl again. They comforted me all that evening until I was well enough to go back to my own house. Then I would worry as I did not want to upset my parents. The cycle was vicious, and I need to break it before it would break me.

There was a huge lesson in that awful day. I knew deep down there was nothing wrong with my heart. I also knew that my body was stronger than I gave it credit for because my body did not let me down and fall into a full-blown panic attack in my relations' house. No, it was cleverer than that, it waited until I had everything ready. My maternal instinct was to protect my baby first and foremost. Then when everything was ready, my body let me fall apart. I was angry at myself for not understanding this and how come the fight or flight waited until I was ready.

I was going to take this head-on, once and for all and gain a healthier life mentally. I started reading some psychology books. I realized for the first time in my life that I could understand all I read. It was never a struggle like schoolwork had once been. It seemed to open my mind and helped me research more into the type of alternative therapies available out there. Fundamentally I am a glass-half-full person. My sole focus was on my health and wellbeing. I believe very much in energy. We are all made of energy and light. I just simply needed to make sure that I worked as hard as I could to keep my energy at a high vibration.

I came across mindfulness and mediation and my life changed yet again. I met a wonderful mindfulness coach in 2012; his name was Will Foster. He was a surfer, personal trainer, and wellbeing coach from the UK. I joined his group of clients and together we put a plan in place. I began journaling my thoughts daily, but the biggest thing that Will taught me was that it was ok "to just be" and sit with our thoughts. I felt like I wanted to run from my thoughts. There were too many of them and they were all over the place. When I sat with them — this took a while to even practice that; I found I immediately began to feel calm. On top of that, he introduced breathing techniques on how to quieten the mind and just reset.

From that, I learnt Shamanic breathing techniques. This involves voluntarily inducing a state of hyperventilation. I felt when I did this, it was a two-finger salute to panic attacks trying to take over.

I was going to show a panic attack that shamanic breathing was, like a Chuck Norris quote "Chuck Norris can kill two stones with one bird". I was going to be Chuck Norris in meditation and wellbeing. I had enough of this!

Slowly, my mindset started to shift. I started gaining control of my breathwork and could even feel my lungs getting stronger. I stopped fighting my feelings. l learnt how to let them be and they passed much more quickly. *Feeling overwhelmed is a call from your soul to slow down to the moment and focus on one thing– Will Foster*

When I started to invest in my mental and physical health, it helped move up another notch on the ladder. I began to meditate longer, from just two minutes initially to now fifteen to twenty minutes. I ate healthier, I enjoyed cooking more, reduced alcohol consumption, began building muscle instead of just wanting to be thin at all costs. After putting the above into motion more frequently, I realized my sleep was better,therefore my mood was equally better. Sometimes as mothers, we think it selfish to think of ourselves, but I call it selfless. It is important to give yourself permission to be the best version of you, to like and, even love yourself, especially after a baby. It's ok to take time for yourself. Life is hard enough without us being harder on ourselves.

On one of my one-to-one meeting with Will, I told him something I always wanted to do but never told anyone as I did not have the self-belief. I told him I wanted to study psychology. I was terrified of failure. I had started a course in fitness training years before and when I failed part of the final exams in anatomy and physiology, I thought that was it for the rest of my life. I put that fear into me. Will asked me a question that to me was life-changing.

He asked me what it would look like on my graduation day — who would be there, what would I wear, what would it feel like. From that moment, my mind had catapulted me into a vision of something I have never experienced before then. I told him the biggest thing for me would be to complete the course and do well in it, to have my parents there and for them to be proud of me, to have my son there to see that it is possible to achieve life-long dreams if you focus on the end result, and to have a party at my home with all my wonderful friends as a thank you to them for always being there and helping me achieve my dreams.

In 2016, my wonderful friend school friend Ailish and I started college together. We were both busy working mom's, full -time jobs, and lots of family commitments. Having Ailish there was great as we worked well together and supported each other with the late night essay writing and the long hours of course work to prepare. College life was exciting, and I looked forward to college every single Thursday evening. There were two modules I absolutely loved. It was Art Therapy and Mindfulness. I had a good practice build-up with the teachings of Will and was working on more personal development rather than looking at it as any other form. It was like I just connected to it when I studied it formally, it all made much more sense. It took me back to that eight-year-old girl and how I was able to help myself back then. I knew this was something I had to do; I wanted to teach this to children. I had a fire in my belly. This is what I was meant to do, and it was my purpose and my goal.

But I had something terribly sad going on in my life. My Mom was extremely ill. Towards the end of my studies, her health had deteriorated so much that she was hospitalized. She was rushed to the hospital one evening. I went straight there and spent the night with her. We thought she would pull out of it as she had before many times, but something was different this time and we knew it. The doctor called me out to the corridor on his early morning rounds. He told me I should contact all the family. His words were "Your Mom is dying". I was numb. How would I tell my sisters, they were so young, they had just started out their lives with their husbands and had small kids to take care of, one of my sisters was expecting and I hated having to tell her. Not to mention my father, who was my rock. How can I tell him his beautiful wife of over fifty years was going to leave him soon? I remember telling one of my sisters, and I cannot remember the conversations after that. All the family congregated at her bedside and she was never alone for the twelve days after that.

I had one last exam to do, and I had no energy. I was sleep -deprived and could hardly even bring myself to think about the exam. I decided that I would take the exam later in the year. I knew I would not be graduating with my colleagues whom we had all shared so much with. I had come home earlier that day from a shift at the hospital. I was so tired that when I came home, all I could do was take my weary self to bed. I slept for a few hours and when I woke, I knew the exam would be on at 6.30 pm. when I got up it was about 5 pm. I had this unbelievable strong urge to go in and sit the exam. It was that higher force again, niggling at me to just go and do it. I was so exhausted that when I even thought about the exam, I could hardly remember how to spell the word psychology, let alone write about it.

I called my best friend Caroline and told her the story. I asked her would she drive me into the exam, wait for me and drive me home again as I was that tired and did not feel comfortable even driving. Caroline said, get up, get dressed, get coffee and she would be there to collect me in fifteen minutes.

I got to the exam and one of the girls Carmel brought me over a prayer for exams which I keep in my wallet every day:

'Loving God, help me as I prepare for my exams especially with those areas of life that are difficult

Help me to study hard and to stay focused

During my exam inspire me to remember all that I need

Give me the ability to express myself clearly

In moments of doubt reassure me that in the end, all will be well.'

I handed over my phone to the invigilator. I explained she might have to take an important call from the hospital. I turned over the questions and the main part of the exam was Kubler -Rosse stages of grief and bereavement. I was talking about the stages of grief as if I knew every one of them, some more than others. Although I still had my mum, just about, I knew the end was near. I had read more on Kubler Rosse's theory of grief as a way of coping with the impending loss we were all going to experience. I wanted to read up as much as I could so that I could understand my feelings and emotions and that it may draw some comfort to my family in their grief.

In these moments of the exam, I could not stop writing. The theories and everything I had learnt was now to the forefront of my mind. I wrote with such deep emotion. I thought of the grief of losing my grandmother when I was twenty-one. It was my first experience of loss and bereavement. I thought of my beautiful sister-in-law, Sarah who was like someone from a Home and Away episode from Australia, who sadly passed away from cancer at age thirty-nine leaving two small beautiful children. She was one of my best friends. I was her age now. She never got to see forty. I was writing for her, for me, for my family, for my friends, for a better life, for loss, for love, for women, for my tribe!

I finished the exam and I felt I wrote everything I could. I felt so relieved to have completed my final exam. I left the college that evening with a sense of pride, knowing I did my absolute best under the extreme condition I was facing. My loyal friend Caroline drove me home that night and I went straight to bed.

The next day it was my shift at the hospital. We were now all congregating, forgetting about which one had which shift. We just all wanted to be there. We drank tea, ate biscuits, and reminisced some funny stories. At one point, my mother opened her eyes and I ran up to the side of the bed and said 'It's me, your favourite daughter', then my sister pushed me out of the way and said 'No, it's not, it's me her', we asked her to blink if once if it was me and twice if it was her. She simply smiled and closed her eyes again.

My mother was deeply spiritual and loved angels. She had an extraordinarily strong faith, so needless to say, there was decades of rosaries said around her bed. My Aunt Noreen handed me the rosary beads and I continued the rosary as a mark of respect to my mother, who was called Mary.

It was Sunday night and I was coming in at midnight to let my other sisters home. I was with my sister-in-law and we took on the night shift together. My sisters reluctantly went home. We were all struggling emotionally. We had young kids to look after in between and little to no sleep. We told them to go home and rest and we would call them if anything changed. Rae and I were getting ready to settle in for the night, one of us on either side of my mother's bed. Rae noticed some changes happening and called the nurses immediately.

They informed me that it was time to hold my mother's hand and let her gently go. I am not sure where the strength came from, but I held it together. I held her hand in mine and stroked her forehead and I kissed my mother goodbye. I told her I loved her and that we would all take care of Pops. I thanked her for being the best mother she could have been, and it was now time for her to go.

My mother passed away that night, holding my hand. It was a huge loss to my entire family, and it hit us hard. My Mum always told me to hold my head up high. I remember those words more today than ever before. I will do that in her honour.

Again, I had to phone my sisters. I asked one of my sisters to phone the others as I just could not. Everyone arrived within a short time and we spent time together as a family one last time. It was beautiful. The pain left my mother's face and she looked like an Angel.

We had the most beautiful funeral for my mother. A full church choir with all her favourite hymns and we gave her the send-off she deserved in true Irish mother style. We fed approximately one hundred people at our family home that day. Just the way our mother would have wanted with everyone going home with something under their arms, scones, brown bread, tarts.

The weeks after that were difficult. We had a lot more time on our hands as we had used all our spare time taking turns visiting our mum in the nursing home. I began my practice of mediations and journaling quite a lot. I was very aware of looking after myself as best I could and to be there for my son, who had also lost his grandmother.

Not long after my mother's death, my marriage also came to an end. It was a very difficult period of my life. One that has taken me on my healing journey, and one I am deeply private about. Not many people knew this had even happened, but my family and friends got me through it. It was moment by moment, hour by hour, day by day. I am happy to say that although Fergal and I are not together, we have nothing but mutual respect for each other. Our son is the most important person in all this. We remain very united and together apart, we are two incredibly good parents. If anyone reading this finds themselves in a situation like this, follow your gut instinct. No one can ever give you the advice on something so personal as a marriage break up. Allow people to support you, reach out to friends, take the help, and trust me, you will need it at times. I was so glad to have this awareness as if I did not have it, I would not have reached out for help. I had the most amazing counsellor who helped me through all this. I would not be half the woman I am today only for Mary. On my last day of counselling, I told Mary I was going to break the code of ethics in counselling. I hugged her to thank her for all she did for me. She hugged me back, both of us holding back the tears. She said, "If you could only see what I see Marie."It was the most comforting, motherly, affectionate words I heard in a long time, and I believed her. I knew I had to go out there and make a life, one that would bring meaning.

In those months, I took great care of myself, and I had some amazing friends — new ones who came into my life for a reason, and close friends who have always been there. My dad had taken up powerlifting competitively at age seventy-eight, he was always fit and strong and never looked (or acted) his age. He suggested maybe I give it a go! So, I did!

My dad trained me at my local gym until I felt fit enough (both mentally and physically). After that, he signed me up to his weightlifting federation. He was a member of the IDFPF 'Irish Drug-free Powerlifting Federation.' I was signed up to compete in a single bench press competition. On the 22nd September 2018, I had my first competition. I bench pressed 47.5kg, and it felt amazing, the adrenaline was pumping, energy was up. My dad had an outstanding lift that day and broke the Irish record for his age and weight. He benched 80kg at age eighty-two! I could not have been prouder. That evening I went home with a pep in my step. That evening we celebrated our victories with a nice dinner out and a glass of wine. Thanks to Pops for always pushing me, I went onto to qualify in the Irish singles lift and somehow managed to qualify for the Europeans single lifts in 2019 in which I came fourth.

I was also studying part-time in the evenings and weekends in mindfulness and creative arts for kids. My lecturer was an amazing teacher. She had such compassion and taught directly from the heart. Learning from Louise Shanagher gave me the skills, belief, and confidence to make the decision to start teaching part-time. I gained great training in promoting positive wellbeing for children in the form of self-compassion. In August 2019, I completed my studies and added to my wellbeing tool kit. I am an accredited Creative Mindfulness & Meditation Kids Practitioner. I teach to children from as young as junior infants. My aim is to promote positive mental health and wellbeing for children to all ages across the board. I am delighted to be accredited to teach in schools, both primary and secondary, as well as my own private practice of group classes.

I am passionate about creating a happier and healthier world for children and young people to grow up in. I passionately believe all children should get the opportunity to learn how to care and promote their positive mental health from an early age. My message is quite simple. I want to introduce positive mental wellbeing into primary schools, making it part of the curriculum to focus on emotional, social and psychological wellbeing. I continue to strive in this and will not stop until I see it through, along with other well-trained and knowledgeable experts in this field. How do you eat an elephant — one bite at a time!

In January 2019, seven months after my mother's passing, I ran my first group of mindfulness classes. I cannot run before I walk. I wanted to gain some first-hand experience with working with children. I wanted to move at the pace that gave me the ability to grow and gain experience. I was also working full-time at the hospital and did not want to take on too much. I spoke to my aunt about my plans. She was so supportive; she was with me at my graduation and is like a second mother to me. She offered to help in my first semester of classes.

My first group of mindful warriors were a joy to teach. I felt a real connection with the children. I could empathize with any little struggles they may have had. And for some kids, they do not have to have struggles; they can choose mindfulness and mediation to learn about being in a state of contentment. We are all capable of so much more than we imagine and so much more than we deserve. So how did I teach these kids?

'You're going to be happy said life, but first I'll make you strong' – Unknown but used by Marie Cronnelly

Teaching mindfulness to children can lead to many positive outcomes, helping them feel calmer and more fulfilled. It improves concentration while empowering them with the tools to deal with stress and anxiety.

I teach the children in small groups to be fully present and by engaging with them We work on breathing techniques to help kids become calm and grounded.

We chat about what mindfulness is and how it can help us. I use a lot of visuals as kids love to see colours and props, including my monkey mind teddy, which shows us how our "monkey mind" is always moving from past, to present to future and how we can control that. I use the mind jar to represent how our busy minds work and how we can calm it down. As we move into the lesson plans, we talk about how feelings are like visitors, they come, and they go. We practice mindfulness of the senses, emotions, and inner value. It is important that we become a good friend to ourselves and I teach many kind, friend-oriented, self-compassion meditations.

The class generally has three main bodies to it:

- Breathwork, i.e. colour breathing, balloon breathing or breathing ball.
- A topic on emotions, with class discussion and worksheets.
- Creative arts, affirmation cards, gratitude tree, mind jars.

We finish up with a gentle guided meditation by me. This is where kids get to lie down on their bean bags, with blankets and just listen while I guide them through a relaxing mediation.

I am incredibly open and honest with the children. I will always mirror what I teach. On the first night I had my class, I asked the children to put their hands up who felt nervous. I included me in that question. I told them that I too was nervous but that these feelings were like visitors coming to visit — they do not stay, they just come, and they go. Discussing emotions and how to handle them at a young age is powerful learning for kids. My contribution to this world is to support young people to navigate their often-scary worlds. As parents, we can learn these skills too and become powerful influencers to our children. I am proud and passionate about my teachings; I have learnt from the best and continue to learn every day.

As we advance through life, too many good souls among us can sometimes lose connection with the awe and wonder that we once knew. I deeply believe that you, me, and everyone alive today has genius within us. Some of us are meant to be leaders in our field. Others are desired to heal or teach the young. All calls on our lives are equal, even though they might look different. No one is above another.

To you and me: do not neglect your brilliance, show your creative side, do not be afraid of it. I feel the main aim of life is not to go deeper into the world but to stop and reclaim all the innocence lost. Become childlike again. The path you take will take you home again. There may be wobbles, bends in the road, hedges to cross and bog drains to jump over. Just put on your wellies, take a deep breath and a big giant leap into it!

Thank you so much for reading my chapter *My Other World*. I am deeply privileged to be able to contribute to this wonderful book and for Galway Simon Community to be the beneficiary of this. Thank you to Sharon for asking me to contribute and for your belief in me.

I have included some testimonials from parents and schools.

Testimonials

It is vitally important that we look after the wellbeing of all our children and we are always looking for new ideas and activities to ensure that our pupils are happy, content, self-aware, confident, assured, and able to deal with any issues and concerns they may encounter. To supplement our Yoga class, we were delighted to welcome Ms. Marie Cronnelly to facilitate a mindfulness workshop with Rang 2 on Wednesday last. The class was utterly amazing and Marie's ability to create an atmosphere of self-awareness, relaxation, reflection, and confidence was indeed special. Probably the most beneficial aspect of Marie's class was her ability to provide the children with coping mechanisms should they feel anxious or concerned. It is our intention to explore the possibility of having Marie return next year to facilitate mindfulness classes with our pupils. Marie, who resides in Athenry, facilitates individual and group workshops and she may be contacted 087 6709520. Further information can be had on Facebook by checking out Marie's Mindfulness and Meditation for Children. **– Joe Kennelly, Principal, Cregmore National School**

Marie's mindfulness and meditation for children is just brilliant! Children are learning through such a fun, relaxed and safe environment how to just be in the moment, to be grounded more and learn to try not to look back or forward! They learn their worries are like clouds and will pass and the most important is that they need to be their own friend before they can be another's! All this and more! Such important life lessons! I highly recommend Marie's classes! My girls were so excited about going every day! **– Joanne Doherty, Athenry**

My two girls of 5+6 just completed a course with Marie, they absolutely loved it and took so much away from it, had lots of fun along the way, Marie was amazing with the children, would definitely recommend it and a big shout out to the lovely Noreen also. – **Brenda Kelly, Athenry**

Charlie just completed his mindfulness course with Marie & had a fantastic experience. So much so that I've him signed up again for the next round. Marie's enthusiasm in this field is so evident. Thanks for everything. - **Paula Shaughnessy – Athenry**

Marie is simply wonderful; my two kiddies a boy (age 9) and girl (age 7) loved everything about this course and do not want to stop going. They had so much fun, felt so comfortable, and they absolutely loved it and cannot wait to go again. Life is so busy for kids these days they really appreciate an hour to relax and unwind, such an amazing place. Thank you so much, Marie, I have two very grounded kids, would absolutely recommend this to anyone I know. – **Karen Ni Donnaile – Headford**

Thank you so much Marie for all the time and effort you put into the zoom classes, mindful packs and for the kindness and understanding to the boys. You have given them the skills to deal with uncertainty and doubt that creeps into all our heads. A work in progress but I am so grateful that they are learning how to be kinder to themselves and to face feelings that none of us like when they do arise. You are a fantastic teacher Marie and a calming presence to all the kids. Enjoy your summer break with your gorgeous boy. – **Shirley Quinn, Galway**

Thank you so much for being a great advocate of Love & Compassion. - **Louise Shanagher, Mindfulness Lecturer, The Mindful Heart**

Marie, from the first time we met in Dublin all those years ago, you gave off a very special vibe. One I don't meet very often. It was said to me, life has some seriously inspiring plans for you. Plans that will unfold the more you get to know who are really are. It's happening and will continue to happen with your mindset. Keep at it..... your destined for great things.– **Will Foster, The Happiness Coach, UK**

https://www.facebook.com/Maries-Mindfulness-Meditation-for-Children

My Journey to Healing
by Norah Coyne

My name is Norah Coyne. I was born and raised by my wonderful Connemara parents, in a small housing estate across the road from the world-renowned Camden Market, in Camden Town, North London. It was not an affluent place then as it is now. It was predominantly Irish. We didn't have much, but we all watched out for each other and it was a lovely place to grow up! We were like one big family, everyone in each other houses, sharing what little we had and growing up together with our trials, tribulations and celebrations.

Camden Lock was a place where buskers, hippies, and all things metaphysical reside. A truly cosmopolitan place many years before it's time. I spent many years hanging out there, learning good and bad! Growing up, swimming in the canal, and listening to the buskers and bands throughout my childhood and early adult years. A place that is still so close to my heart today!

My beginning did not quite go according to plan! I was born on the hottest day of the year which was of great discomfort to my poor mother and made her quite ill. My birth although uncomfortable she said it felt ok at the beginning, she just felt a little weak! A few minutes later, when the nurses examined me, they noticed a cyst half the size of my head, on the back of my skull. I was rushed away from my mother to an incubator in intensive care, where I spent the next few weeks.

My poor mother was distraught! She had no idea what was going on and had to be sedated. (It was many years later that I realised that the lack of attachment and bonding then, was the cause of some of my insecurities later in my life). The priest was called and my poor father and his uncle who were waiting were told, "you have to name your daughter now! We need to perform the last rites". They did not know what to do!

As my mother was sedated, and I was so ill, they decided on Norah as both of my grandmothers were strong women called Norah, so that was the choice. I am sure that the name they gave me that day also gave me a strength that would be with me forever. Norah means honour and in Arabic, Fire and Shining Light. I truly feel they blessed me that day with my name.

Throughout the next few months, I improved and was looked after by the wonderful Great Ormond Street Hospital, where my poor mother would have to hold me in her arms as they lanced open my head to drain it every week. Her determination and loving care got us through. Although she did say I cried constantly for six months, God bless her! She said I only stopped crying if she kept singing a Gaelic lullaby. That it must have been my first connection with the healing power of sound. I know now that it was the sound and vibration of her voice helping me heal. I still use that same lullaby today to calm some of the special needs children I work with.

People ask if I remember my birth. I explain to them that I just always had a knowing that while we were apart in that incubator, I was being held safely by someone or something who I later realised was my guardian Angel Sarah who I still work with today!

Life was pretty happy after that and I don't remember any visions or connections until I was around four years old. I so wanted a black and white fluffy push around dog from Santa

Claus, I would ask him every night before I went to sleep. Then a couple of days before Christmas, I was playing up in the bedroom and I kept hearing, 'The dog is here for you. You have the dog, the black and white one.' I didn't pay any heed to it at the time, but when Christmas Day came, it was there! I didn't notice any other signs, although I am sure they were around me! My life just seemed normal until I was sixteen. I was a bit of a wild free spirit, always out enjoying life, not a care in the world. It was then that my favourite uncle Johnny and my close friend Alan died. I was distraught for a long time.

Johnny was my mum's favourite brother who was living with us, so really I lost her that day too for a while as she couldn't cope with his loss. It took her a very long time to come to terms with it and through no fault of her own, I had no mother to help me through the early stages of grief. When Alan died in very tragic circumstances a few weeks later, I just couldn't cope and went off the rails completely.

It took me a few years to come back to a new normal which was when around the age of twenty-one partly by chance partly by accident, I had my first taste of sound healing. It was an amazing journey really! I was in London down at Camden Lock. It was there I first came across healing techniques in my earlier years. There was everything from energy healing, to palmistry and tarot readings to witchcraft and healing from most parts of the globe. An amazing place to be! It was a world that intrigued my friends and me from an early age. We were like children in a sweet shop, in awe of some of the things we saw and tried out and amazed at the weird and wonderful people who travelled through. Although I did not actually realise how important it would be in my life, it was there that I first found the wonder that is Intuitive and Vibrational Sound Healing.

I was twenty-one years old and as I browsed through the market alone, I was searching for something in life, I didn't know what it was. My life wasn't great and I was confused about where I wanted to be or who I wanted to be, I was trying to find myself, after losing my uncle Johnny and Alan. I just couldn't find my way back. The effect of their losses had stayed with me for such a long time.

I was walking by the stalls and a sound was drawing me towards it, a bit like a pied piper. I looked ahead and it was there I saw a vibrantly dressed lady giving sessions with Tibetan Healing bowls and I was very drawn to the music. I don't know why but I explained more in a few minutes to her than I told anyone else in years. To this day I still believe it was the vibration of the sound that drew me to her to help me that day.

She sat me down on the chair and started to first play the sound around me, above my head down through my aura and all around the air that surrounded my body. I could feel tingling everywhere. It was as if things were unfolding and releasing without having to say anymore. The tears streamed down my face. It was such a relief to let them out. It was if she knew where to place each bowl to get the best and the worst out of me. The heaviness was leaving; my body felt so light and free and at ease.

After the session, I noticed she was selling bowls and I asked her if I could buy one, she told me to play with them and that I would know instinctively the one that was meant for me which I did. When I asked her about the bowl, she explained to me, it was for the throat chakra and would help me "speak my truth". At the time I had no idea what she meant, but found out many years later exactly what it would be! I was releasing what no longer served me and leaving space for the new.

Within a few weeks of that session, I changed my job and my outlook on some parts of my life, left my relationship and started to get back in touch with my feelings and sensations that were dull for so long, my wildness reignited that day and stayed with me for good and for bad, as I explored life to find out where I was meant to be. There was definitely something different about me that day. I think I knew in my heart I was never going to be the same again as I felt so different, lighter, freer and in tune with what was going on in my life, I felt like I was 'more me' even though I didn't quite know what that was.

Throughout the time I had the bowl, I didn't really use it much and had it on a shelf in my bedroom as a reminder of that day as I never dreamed I would be able to do what that lady in Camden did for me that day. Then as if all of a sudden, I started to let go of fear, especially the fear of being left alone that I had felt for a very long time, which I still believe originally stemmed from that early detachment from my mother. I started to come out of my shell, trying and learning therapies, it was as if my real life's journey had just begun.

I decided it was time to return to Connemara for some reconnection with my beautiful grandmothers as the love they both showed me was a love like no other. The connection I had with both of them in different ways was so powerful. The feeling that to them everyone is a perfect being of light no matter what you have done or not done, the pure unconditional love that surrounds you forever without judgement, without having to give anything in return. It was during this visit many moons ago that I met my partner Matt. We had a brilliant time together while I was in Connemara and it didn't hurt that my mother and both grandmothers loved him! When it was time to leave, Matt decided to move to London with me, we have been together ever since and the rest, as they say, is history!

Throughout this I always had a knowing I was being drawn somewhere and decided to return to Camden to learn the ways of the Tarot and through the years since then, have lived through most of them. That journey which, I can truly say, made me the person I am today. I think I have lived all of the cards in the tarot many times. It was like a mirror image of my soul, the Tarot showing me and making me live my innermost fears and showing me where to go next. Believe me when I say that the Tarot is no fool. It really opened up my true self both the dark and the light to make me face life head-on and find my path! This journey took me from trying out different things, some that suited me, some that didn't, some good, some bad, to the ones that took me to receiving and eventually learning the many therapies that I have worked with in my life up until now. Low and behold, while working with the Tarot which is a vibration, I came across an article on musical tones for the major arcana in Tarot and started to use those tones within my healing work and readings.

I think it was getting me ready for the journey I was going to embark on. The universe was giving me these tones for my healing toolbox to use when the time was right. Over the next couple of years, I was not really intending to work fully as a therapist, it was more something I was starting to love as it became part of my being.

I was working in a very highly paid but stressful job in London. Around every corner, friends or family would need a Tarot Reading or a course that interested me would come up as if by chance or synchronicity. The biggest synchronicity came when I was in a car accident. My sister Bridget was driving and her little girl Mary Ann was in the child seat behind me. We were parked at the traffic lights when there was an almighty bang and we were sandwiched between two cars. Thankfully, we were not seriously hurt. My injury was the worst, which was whiplash and a knee injury. Although I was still able to work, due to the pain and restriction, I had physio for a while but I didn't seem to be improving. A friend told me about a wonderful therapist called Julie Ann so I went to her for two sessions and I have never looked back.

As I told Julie Ann my story, she handed me a leaflet for the Academy of Natural Health for An Introductory Massage Course; she told me she thought it would really help me find my direction. I was so drawn to it and didn't know why. At the time I didn't even think it was possible I would be able to do it, so I left the leaflet on the kitchen table and went to bed. When I came down in the morning, the money for the course was on the leaflet. Matt remembered my birthday was the following week and left the money there for me. I knew then it was fate!

I was so nervous going to the course. I knew nothing about massage. The teacher had paired me with a Japanese girl called Zuki. We were taught to do a leg and back massage. As I massaged Zuki she was so relaxed, she fell asleep, I felt so connected to her during the work, it was as if her body was a map of emotions and I was being drawn to certain places that seemed to relax her more. In the background, Tibetan Bowl Music was playing.

After the class I said to the teacher, "Did you see how quickly she fell asleep?" She giggled, I wondered why and she said, "Norah, she just got off the plane from Japan this morning, I don't want to burst your bubble, but she's probably jetlagged!" We laughed and laughed, then she said, "Norah as I watched you, it was as if the two of became one, as you flowed with the sound and massage, I noticed that your breaths and auras were intertwined and your connection became one." I knew she was right, that's just how I felt.

I just knew it was for me, so I enrolled in the full Diploma there and then which consisted of many different types of massage, healing, sound, shamanic work and community healing circles. It was life-changing for me, it was the last part of the puzzle to help me walk on my path of healing and vibration. I had found my vocation in life!

I was very drawn to my bowl again and started to play it around my throat chakra. It was amazing the way my creativity started to flow, my throat chakra was unblocked, my truth was releasing, I was speaking my truth. Now I knew what it meant!

Over the next while we decided to move back to Ireland to be near our parents, but I still travelled far and wide training in different Sound Therapy and Healing Courses, training with some of the best mentors in the world. It was always the sound I was drawn back to. With every course I grew, with every treatment I received healing. It was working on my physical body, my mind and my heart. It did more for me than any other therapy I have ever had. It was as if I had found my medicine, as if it was what I should always have done. It was something I couldn't go back from, it worked so well with the way I work intuitively. It tells me so much when I work with sound on someone and the results are amazing.

After thirteen years here in Connemara, I sadly lost my beautiful mother Mary to the light. The loss of my mother is something even to this day is very hard to bear. She was very ill for her last two years on this planet where more and more she began to love the connection of touch and therapies. She loved me using tuning forks on her weary back and legs, she was too frail for anything else near her transition and would ask me often for a few minutes of energy work. It gave us the connection that I thought we had lost. It was a true bonding as if we were being brought together again to make up for that time we had lost when I was born, but this time I was the minder and she was the one needing to be minded! I was so honoured I was able to work with her in her last few hours as she transitioned into the light!

Within weeks of the funeral, I had a serious meltdown. The heart of my world was gone. My stability, my rock, the woman who brought me into this world and cared for me so much was gone. It was something I could not bear! My body just fell apart. I could not sleep, could not eat. My lungs became very weak. It was the grief, and it was at its worst for two months. Sadness and depression had set in. There was no one who could understand the way my mum did. It was the worst I have ever felt in my life.I pretended to those outside I was coping but really, I was not! Then out of the blue, my cousin's wife called me and told me she was thinking of me. She had seen a course in Leitrim about making your own singing bowl. It was a circle of women, working on the shamanic path, spending three days together to birth our own singing bowl. It just seemed like it came at the right time, so three of us decided to go and see what it was all about.

Well, if you want to release everything back to the bone, laugh, cry, scream, shout, and release throughout the three days, it was the place to be! We started in ceremony and the then picked our sheet of metal. For three days we hammered the metal, then placing it in the fire, on the earth, in the water, in the air. We worked with all the elements, then sang, and held each other's energy and started again and again and again. We sang together, ate together, played sound instruments together, until eventually after all the tears, stories and laughter of women from all over the world were shared, we were each left with a beautiful bowl. When it came to the last part of the ceremony, I placed my bowl in the fire for the last time.

As we sat singing in circle remembering my mother, the shape of a heart came into the bowl, we were so excited when we saw the sign from my mother. She was letting me know that it was ok to let her go! As the bowl cooled, the heart disappeared and I knew this would now be my bowl and she would be with me as I worked with it. The sound and vibration of the bowl is different from any other bowl I have so I know it is truly meant for me!

What Is Sound Healing?

Well, the easiest way I can describe the amazing work that Sound Healing allows me to do is that it is like giving your body and soul an NCT or Tune-Up. Working in the present moment but also helping you clear past patterns and blockages as well as releasing the fluidity within you to follow your future path!

Intuitive Sound Healing can be done in many ways, in a meditation and healing environment, where everyone in the room will receive the specific frequency tune-ups they need, for couples, groups, one to one or specialised works such as corporate or wellness events, healing days and retreats, in schools and festivals. It has even been done at funerals

To understand how I work with these tools, try and imagine your body is a piano and all the ailments, emotions, thoughts, and imbalances from this dimension or any other are the piano keys which are 'out of tune.' When the vibration of sound flows through your cells and tissues, those piano keys are returned and rebalanced, bringing you back to being you.

It is a beautiful non-invasive healing session guided by universal spiritual energy and frequencies that help you get balance in your daily life, as we are all living as part of life's symphony of frequencies and the rebalancing it brings is awesome. It is not just about the spiritual aspect with sound, it is also made up of energy vibrating at different frequencies which correspond to certain musical notes.

All things in nature vibrate to sound, light, and colour. (That is why I chose to work with them). The organs, glands, and cells and tissues of our bodies vibrate at their own specific frequencies corresponding to these musical notes. (So for example, a healthy heart which would vibrate at the frequency of the F note so if you played a tuning fork, Tibetan bowl, or sang mantras in the frequency of F, they would energise or calm the heart and emotions). Frequencies affect everything about us, therefore they can be used to heal and balance too!

When your body is in perfect health and all the parts are vibrating to the correct note, your body is playing beautiful music so think of the different body parts as musical instruments all vibrating at their own unique sound. When the bodies parts are playing the right note and vibrating in harmony, energy flows through your healthy body and soul like a river or stream, through a network of meridians and chakras (like trains travelling through stations). However, stress, negative emotions, and thoughts, even the foods we eat can restrict the flow.

When the energy gets blocked, the body part where the blockage is can no longer play the right note. Although we may not be able to hear this, the body feels this and will display symptoms to let us know when something is wrong and that it needs to be brought back in tune. The powerful sound vibrations of sound instruments, including the voice, can be used to clear these blockages that are affecting the body's flow of energy and restructure the flow.

The instruments I use, (Singing Bowls, Gongs, Tuning forks, for example), work along the same meridians and points as acupuncture, so a Tuning Fork Treatment is like Acupuncture without the needles or intrusion into the skin. When the correct instrument is used on the organ or chakra that is out of harmony, that area will raise its vibration to that of the fork by the process of entrainment. If an area is depleted, the energy will rise, if it is over-energised it will relax bringing rebalance back into the area.

It is ideal if you are a little nervous about, intrusion into your space, as you can remain fully clothed and it is also very gentle but powerful without pain, or manipulation involved. As the sounds flow through your body, your cells start to pulsate, resonate, and interact with the powerful vibrations, thus awakening the life energy of the cells and returning you to health and harmony.

Some Of The Wonderful Benefits Of Sound Therapy

It increases your physical energy and releases the wonderful "pain-reliving" 'feel good' endorphins, helping you reach a deep state of relaxation and induces the alpha–theta brain states associated with healing.

It also helps synchronise your mind-heart-body rhythms and opens and rebalances your chakras and organs.

Sound improves your meridian flow, encouraging expansion of your creative flow, which gives you clarity and improved concentration and assists the removal of toxins and encourages soft tissue healing.

Harmonising the emotional and physical bodies, integrates the left and right brain thought patterns and supports healthy circulation of the bodily fluids and immune system function.

Sound Healing is immensely powerful and can move molecules, rearrange realities, and penetrate any substance. It moves four times faster in water than in air, and as the human body is 70% water, that makes us perfect resonators for this therapy. Sound waves can produce changes in the autonomic, immune, endocrine, and neuro-peptide systems of the physical body. Just think about it — Doctors use sound to treat kidney stones by non-invasively focusing a harmonic frequency on the stones. Kidney stones are a special type of crystal whose atoms vibrate at a specific frequency. The focused sound waves interact with the atoms of the kidney stones, causing the stones to vibrate so quickly that the stones disperse and dissolve. Sound is also used in Ultrasound on a mother's belly to see how healthy her baby is doing. There are many ways that you may have already used sound in your life and not even realised it.

What Is It I Actually Do?

"I truly believe everyone has the power to self-heal and follow their own life's purpose; sometimes we just need a little help." My intention is and always has been to help you rebalance your inner wellness with a truly holistic approach and help you to help yourself on your own self-healing path.

My work is guided uniquely and intuitively to whatever you specifically need at each particular visit by working with a combination of all things vibrational together with my intuition, so that would include my Sound Healing Therapy 'toolbox' where I use specific sound instruments of various frequencies, such as Gongs, Tibetan and Crystal Bowls, Drums, Chimes, Rain sticks and Voice (through meditation or mantra). I include the other vibrational tools I work with such as Crystals, Colour, Tarot and Energy Work; at all times guided by my intuition and where your energy and my spirit guides are taking me to enable you to get the best you possibly can from your treatment.

My focus is on rebalancing your emotional, psychological, spiritual, physical, social, mental, and superficial aspects to assist you in getting to a place to empower you on your own healing path. This can work on your present situation, past situations, as far back as your past lives and removal of blockages to help future situations.

Just for a moment think of when you are listening to upbeat or cheery music, you want to dance and smile, or when listening to deep songs, our emotions come into play, then think of yourself leaning against a large speaker, and heavy metal or punk rock like the Sex Pistols is blaring out! Each of these different frequencies brings different aspects of vibration to your body so your emotions may flare or calm or release depending on what frequency is going through your energy body. Let us say you have a headache. A sound can be played that will override the pain brainwaves. Or you are in a bad mood after a poor night's sleep. Playing a relaxing song might lift your spirits and help you forget you are aggravated. Ironic when I look back now, that while I was lost when I was sixteen, I was a punk rocker and the sweet sounds of Bob Marley and Kris Kristofferson balance and warm my heart now!

Intuitive sound healing can vastly improve many areas of your life, including emotional, psychological, and mental health, social development, cognitive and motor functioning. I have achieved amazing results and interaction with sound in my work in the special needs centres from children to adults with cerebral palsy to autism. The reaction from some of the children and adults is magical. The way they interact and connect with the sound is something that has brought so much joy! The cognitive and physical way our brains and bodies respond to sound is something that must be experienced to really understand how wonderful it is.

I run Sound Baths from ages 0 to 100+ for the general public, for corporate and wellness events, for couples, and one of the ways I especially love is for mothers-to-be and parent and babies. It's amazing to see when I work with mothers to be how the babies are tuning into the vibrations in the womb before they are even born in the physical word. The connection here between mother and child is a feeling that I can only describe as "miraculous" as they both receive the same vibrations but each one inside the other receive exactly what they need. The babies can be calm or dancing around the belly but almost always very responsive and the mummy relaxing and chilling out. When the babies are born, their births are usually very calm and chilled and their reaction to sound and vibration from their first breath is so lovely the way they can interact so naturally.

A sound bath for a group of adults will send the sound to everyone in the room each receiving something very different. Some will be completely relaxed and feel an out of body experience, others may just sleep, and for some the vibration will stay in certain areas until the blockage has dispersed. Everyone's story is different, everyone's journey is their own. I am just a facilitator they are allowing the journey, they are allowing me to do what I do, I have the tools and the training, but they are allowing me to travel with them on a small part of their journey to take them where they need to be.

I work with stress issues, such as anxiety, depression, self-esteem and Inner Child work, healing circles, empowerment days and Moon Mna Divine Feminine Monthly Groups, incorporating sound and healing as its expansive nature can travel beyond borders to get into the real issue sometimes without having to actually talk about it at all. It's as if the sound flows through to the source, shakes it all up, to rebalance, realign, replenish and refresh to enable you to get to a point to restart from, sometimes without even have to speak a word.

These are just a few cases (names changed for privacy) to give you an idea of how Intuitive Sound Healing helps physical aspects of your being.

Josephine's Story (Thyroid Imbalance)

When Josephine, a working mother of three came to me, she had recently completed iodine treatment for a thyroid imbalance and was in an awful way. She was very lethargic and found it hard to get out of bed. It was very difficult for her as she used to run 10k every week and she wasn't even strong enough to take the children to school. She was very down, tired all the time and her mood swings were erratic, one moment there were tears another anger. She found it very hard coping, she was desperate for help. She had already discussed it with her doctor and they had both agreed it was the Thyroid that was the main cause. Within hours of the first session, Josephine's energy was better. She took the children to school the following morning and walked half a kilometre. By the fourth session her Thyroid had rebalanced and the doctor had reduced her medication by a quarter. She was so happy. She continues to go from strength to strength and a year later, her Thyroid medication is still the lowest it has ever been. Josephine still comes once every few months as she enjoys the relaxation she feels from the sound.

Michael's Story (Severe Autism)
Michaels diagnosis is severe autism and was in one of the special needs schools I attend on a frequent basis. When I was asked to work with him, we didn't quite know how it would go so I brought in a selection of tools. I thought I would play them all one at a time to gauge his interest and reaction before I worked on him. The staff were not sure how he would react. I sat on a chair next to him and showed him the tools. As I played one of the bowls he reached out and put his fingertips against the bowl and was feeling the vibration of it. Every time I played the bowl, the same thing happened. He had no interest in the other ones. Then I did the same with the tuning forks and the drums. I was able to work out then which instruments he was comfortable with. When I started playing the drum, I watched his fingers and he was playing the same rhythm on his knee, it was something I had never seen before. I handed him my spare drum and he did the same. We realised then that Michael's sessions needed to be with him interacting and playing with the instruments not just

receiving them. I worked with Michael for months and every time he saw me, he would come right in and play. The principal was amazed. He truly loved the sound, they said he was so calm in the school the weeks he had his sound sessions which were obvious to see. They only stopped when Michael finished school to move on to an Adult Facility.

Teresa's Story (Severe Rheumatoid Arthritis)
Teresa was one of my favourite clients. Sadly she has since passed into the light. She was someone very special, suffering for many years from severe rheumatoid arthritis, so much so that her chest was severely congested and she could hardly walk. The damage was advanced. Her legs and were so swollen and painful, she needed help to walk. She first came to me for massage and it was then that I introduced her to Tuning forks as they were much less intrusive on her feet than massage. She felt much lighter in the feet afterwards and her nose also started dripping and her chest started to clear a little. The next time she came in she asked me to try them on her chest. We used the bone frequency forks and the immune forks which worked really well for her. Teresa came to me whenever the congestion or pain would get too much for her, either monthly or weekly over a period of about a year. She always found tremendous relief. It was one of the treatments she could do as she was so ill that most medications made her ill and could not be prescribed to her. The way the forks opened the fluidity and energised the meridians was amazing.

I hope you enjoyed reading my story and that our paths may cross one of these days! Blessings and Light from my heart to yours, Norah x

Testimonials

Norah's sound baths are the best in the business. I am obviously biased! I have been to a few others! When Norah performs, it is pure bliss. An energetic reset for my body, mind, and soul. I feel lighter like I am cloud walking, so relaxed, I feel physical blockages shift; see the colours of my chakras in my mind's eye vividly as she plays and can think clearly by the end.

Sound can shift frequencies from low energy of guilt and fear to higher vibrations of love and joy, but when it's done from a level of love and passion from Norah, it's even more enriching. It's how Norah plays the instruments and reads the energy of each individual and the room as a whole that makes her extra special. I am so am blessed and lucky to have Norah in my life. – **J. Maloney, Galway**

It is just a delight and pleasure to work alongside Norah. We started our Yoga sound bath events for pregnant mom's, their partners and grandparents and parents and babies two years ago inspired to try something different! The feedback has been so positive. Combining yoga with the sound bath feels like time stops and all are held within the beautiful sounds, frequencies, and vibrations of this unique experience. Norah is very attuned to the baby inside and outside, so sounds are at a safe level for their sensitive ears. Inducing deep relaxation for all with an interactive experience for babies which is truly magical. – **Penny Jones Yoga**

We absolutely loved Norah from the first time we met her. We attended our first sound bath with my husband when I was pregnant with our son. The sound bath was one of the highlights of my pregnancy. Beside the fact that we came out of the experience being so relaxed and recharged, we never felt so connected to the bump. We were overwhelmed by all the movements and reactions from the baba during the sound bath. Norah had that energy that I cannot really explain. It was just magical. It was such a special morning and it felt like the time has stopped for a few hours and nothing else mattered but soothing sounds and the connection to the baby and to each other with my husband. When the baby was born, we noticed straight away how much comfort he found in different sounds and music, so there was no question attending Norah's sound bath again. Most babies were relaxing and sleeping during the experience, but my boy was way too curious and engaged, could not take his eyes of Norah or the musical instruments. Norah was so kind and patient letting him touch all the equipment's and showed him everything he had an interest in. I really did not want the morning to end–it was such a great bonding time for us. He was so relaxed afterwards slept through most of the afternoon.

We attended another sound bath when my son was a bit older and that is what the real fun was for him, I think. He was obsessed with the ocean drum and gong and could not wait to try all out. Of course, Norah was happy to let us try anything and shared her knowledge about the instruments which made the event even more interesting and special. Norah is such a beautiful and humble person; it was a privilege to take part in her sound baths and I would recommend her highly to anyone. – **Emese Juhasz**

I first came across Norah Coyne and Sound Baths when I was coming to the end of my yoga journey (pregnancy and baby) with Penny Jones. I went along to it, not knowing what to expect, but it was a nice way to mark our last class with the girls who had become friends over the past months. I found it very therapeutic, allowing me to switch off in a room that was full of under eight-month-olds. My daughter was fascinated by all the sounds and loved being in the bowl at the end, where Norah vibrated sounds around her. My second meeting with Norah was when I was forty weeks plus ten days pregnant with my son. I attended the Pregnancy Sound bath, again hosted with Penny Jones. I was amazed at the baby movements as the sounds circled the room around me. We were both relaxed and ready for our birth story by the end of such a wonderful session. I returned with baby John a few months later to the mother and baby Sound Bath and he was amazed by the sounds he was hearing, this time he could hear them on the outside. Now, pregnant with my third baby. I yet again had a new experience with Norah and her sound bath, this time via Zoom, even though Norah was many miles away from us, we all allowed ourselves to drift into the sounds that were being created. Everybody needs something like this to switch off from busy home and work lives and have some 'me' time. It leads to clearer minds, more productivity and happier in one's self. Norah is a wonderful lady who has a very calming presence and I recommend a sound bath experience to all. – **Roisin O'Reilly**

The day we were with Norah, was one of the most beautiful days I remember in my babies first year. An endearing smile comes to my face when I remember Mateo touching the bowls, full of excitement and curiosity and looking around searching the origin of those soft and vibrant sounds. I think the atmosphere she created was special, a very cosy and beautiful space. Norah was really kind and adapted perfectly the sound, the volume and the rhythm for the babies, showing them the instruments, letting them touch and experience the different instruments and sounds and feeling the vibrations of the Tibetan bowls, even inside a big one, it was a unique, magical experience! – **Marta Munoz**

My daughter Ellen and I attended a Sound Bath for babies with Norah in February. I was not sure what to expect but had been recommended by a friend. It was the loveliest morning. It was so relaxing. My daughter Ellen loved the different sound and she especially enjoyed being placed in the bowls and feeling the vibrations. She had the most peaceful nap after the session. I would highly recommend the sound bath as a special time out with your baby. – **Tara Kelly**

Norah's sound baths sustained me through lots of personal challenges. They were always a place of release, a space to breathe and be, knowing that all was well and that I was surrounded by loving support. Norah is a skilled practitioner in so many disciplines and combines many practices seamlessly, her use of gongs, singing bowls and chimes always managed to reset my energies, leaving me feeling both relaxed and refreshed! – **Brenda Kenny**

Norah is my go-to person for healing work. I always feel grounded leaving her Sound Healing or Crystal bed Sessions, grounded and ready to go back into a busy life feeling present and intentional! – **Pat Divilly, Galway**

Norah Coyne
Sound Healing Therapist-Healing Intuitive-Energy & Vibration Practitioner-Intuitive Bodywork-Angel & Tarot Reader, Energy EFT (Emotional Freedom Technique), Reiki, Rahanni & IET (Integrated Energy Therapy) Master, Bio Energy Therapist, Sacral Abdominal Therapist, Clinical & Spiritual Aromatherapist & Reflexologist, Aura Soma Colour Therapist, Yoga & Meditation Teacher, Healing and Empowerment Workshops & Retreat Facilitator, Moon Mna & Community Healing Circles, Life Skills Consultant

I can be contacted via www.connemarahealing.net
Tel: 0870563411
Facebook: connemarahealingintuitivemassageenergyandsound

When I Let Go Of What I Am, I Become What I Might Be
by Stephanie Dowling-Folan

It all began the summer of 2006. I remember well what life was like for me, a busy mom to a two-and-a-half-year-old toddler, a physical therapy business on the rise, working two jobs, gym training most days, and being a part of the underage provincial youths rugby team set up, which involved home and away travel, but it was how I liked it. Life for me was always high adrenaline, fast-paced, busy, hardworking, one of giving all the time, but from a mindset of perfectionism, never being enough and always aiming to please. For me, I was driven by a need to achieve, not from a place of ego, but one of self-belief in lack, a need to fit in and be accepted, a drive to belong. In my earlier years, I loved to be active. I played squash at inter-provincial level, was one of the first women in the Military Police of the reserve defence forces and set up a personal training company when they were probably unheard of in Galway. I also went on to play rugby at inter-provincial and then international level, proudly the second out-half from Galway playing on an Irish team!

When I retired due to injury, I went on to coach rugby at the University College Galway, then my local team Galwegians (where it all began), followed by the Connacht Women's Team. Life was always full of schedules, training sessions, places to be, people to meet; there were never enough hours in the day. Burnout was surely never going to be too far away. It's strange now looking back at a time when everything seemed normal enough, but in hindsight, I was operating on an empty cylinder, eating on the run, broken, light sleep but that is all I had ever known, so I didn't see it coming. That is the thing with most disease, symptoms are "always" there, but we are just too distracted, too busy, maybe even sub-consciously not wanting to recognise when something feels off but ploughing ahead anyway until we cannot anymore. That is when we must sit up and listen to not only what our bodies but also our heart is conveying to us.

It started very slowly and fatigue being my first symptom, but for someone who never stopped, it was one I definitely noticed. It was tiredness at bone level. I was pushing through, but I felt different somehow, not myself, followed by three more symptoms, body itch and pain, night sweats and nausea, all which stuck with me for seven more months before I received a medical diagnosis.

It wasn't that I didn't try to source the root of my issues, I just about knew my local GP. I had never been sick, so on his advice, I went to see several consultants and doctors, had numerous tests, scans, ultrasound — you name it, I did it. I even briefly tried the complementary and herbal route but to no avail at that time. Interestingly, it was suggested that I try an anti-depressant that might help with my stomach issues as they could not find any medical reason for my symptoms and weight loss. I was gone too far, and my body was about to 'wake me up' so I was going down that road, whether I wanted to or not.

Finally, an acutely inflamed right eye was about to change the course of my life in ways beyond my wildest comprehension. I felt bombarded by all that was happening to me, rushed to my ophthalmologist, more tests, more consultants, and a worried expression that something more sinister was underlying all these symptoms. My world as I knew it was about to change forever.

I was travelling to the North with the U–15 Youths Connacht Rugby team and we had left very early that morning. I had been up for hours earlier, with a niggling pain in my back that made me vomit but thought nothing of it. By the time we arrived at the hotel reception, I was deteriorating. The pain was starting to slowly spread, down my legs up my arms and the vomiting was incessant. An urgent visit to the local A&E, pain injections and medication that I could not keep down, with the advice to return to Galway ASAP. I needed full medical intervention.

The following hours I will never forget. The pain turned out to be acute peripheral neuropathy. How I described it to people is like somebody had my finger in a wall socket and I was being electrocuted. It was becoming impossible to function. When I arrived at A&E in Galway, I was not able to stand. I was assessed on my knees, the pain was so unbearable. Nobody knew what to do, there was no diagnosis. Morphine followed for the next seven days with a hospital stay that involved many tests and no decisive conclusions. Finally, a new consultant, just back from the US, who had just started in Galway, met with me, looked at all my symptoms, and even though every single blood test was negative, the words: Wegener's Polyangiitis Granulomatosis was diagnosed. What on earth was that?

I felt relieved I at least had a reason for all my symptoms now. Something was wrong with me and like my attitude with everything in life at that time, I will get it sorted and get back to normality. Little did I know the life I was getting back to, was going to be a quite different one!

What followed for the next twelve months, was medical treatment, that resulted in immediate early menopause, my beautiful hair fell out, my body blew up with steroid weight gain, my daily regime of sixteen to twenty-two tablets per day, was one I had to get used to, but I was clueless and trusted the only people who were able to help me at that time. My love of exercise was temporarily halted, my sleep pattern involved one to two hours per night due to the excessively high level of steroids, but I continued to function daily, as I was self-employed. I choose my own work hours, my daughter needed looking after and I was ever so grateful for her grannies and extended family who loved and looked after her when I was unable.

What it did give me though was something I didn't have before and that was TIME — time to reflect, time to think about what was happening, time to listen to that 'voice in my head' that kept nudging me to really look at what was going on in my life. Something did not feel right about all of this. It was like watching a movie of myself and as the director, I wanted to shout "CUT" and change the script!

Maybe it was those feelings of the lack of control to what was happening, the uncomfortable thought that I was only treating symptoms, which did help for sure, but not the root cause which was always active. Autoimmune conditions you are told have no known cause, no known cure and you'll live with it for the rest of your life. I couldn't, wouldn't accept that diagnosis. It just made no sense to me. My body was talking to me, it was in a deep state of unease, (dis-ease) if you like, and to me, had no known cause YET, no known cure YET was to be the catalyst on the road I was about to embark upon.

Mainstream medicine is committed to improving an outcome for a person, through what is best available at any particular time, chemistry, science and pharmacology, but anything outside of that box is considered 'alternative' and not much research or documentation was available on the power of the bigger picture. That being said, disease does not have a single cause. Many factors in our biology, psychology and social environments need to be looked at if we are to find balance and harmony on the mental, emotional, physical and spiritual levels.

The knowledge I have gained over the past few years has allowed me to view health and wellness, even life itself with a whole new perspective. So many insights have brought a new awareness, a very conscious one to help me compassionately and with empathy break down the narrative, I held around my own life.

They say when the student is ready, the teacher will appear and the following months after that diagnosis, I found myself for hours in front of the computer, reading anything I could get my hands on regarding autoimmune disease, researching medical and scientific sites, books that could give me any indication how to fix my broken body. I was on a mission and determined to not live my life with a LABEL; the idea of that was just not acceptable to me. It was while on one of those research missions, I found the endearing Louise Hay book, *You Can Heal Your Life*, which was to be the start of my journey into the world of mind and body connection, self-love and self-care, and the realisation that this is MY body, which is mirroring back to me the 'story' of what's going on inside my mind, one I was about to unravel.

I had never seen the physical body as anything other than a lump of flesh and bones that worked without my conscious intervention, certainly the idea of energy flow, soul or spiritual awareness, mind–body connection was alien to me. Call it fate or divine intervention, I'm not quite sure myself, but finding myself in the world of Bio-Energy, Reiki, Kinesiology, Homeopathy, Meditation, Crystal Healing, Yoga, Childhood and Ancestral Healing, Cellular Memory, Hidden Mind and Sound Therapy, Shamanic work, Essential oils, Acupuncture & Traditional Chinese Medicine, and eventually supplementation, a whole new realisation was dawning on me.

I was walking around in a bubble, with no real awareness of who I was or what I was doing. It was 'mindless' living. I functioned without thinking, not realising that even though I thought I was in control, I was in fact living out a paradigm handed down to me from generations past. Nothing changes without action, and despite all the knowledge I had accrued, putting it into practice wasn't always going to be so easy. I still struggle with shifting old beliefs, emotions and patterns that have been ingrained within my psyche, waiting for me to become aware of their existence and willingness to let them go. This is a process, one not to be rushed because we have somewhere to get to, no, far from that, it's an awakening, an awareness of the loss of something so precious, that the journey back to it, is actually the real purpose of our life here, the connection back to the 'essence' of who we truly are. To do that, we need support, wisdom, empathy, non-judgment, and unconditional love. I had to start with myself first before I could allow these processes to become a part of the work practises I continue with today. One of those practices, which I will talk about in this section is Acupuncture and Traditional Chinese Medicine, a modality, thousands of years old, that I still feel privileged to learn and practise every day.

Acupuncture is one of the oldest forms of medical treatment in continuous use in Asia for more than 5,000 years and has gained general acceptance in the Western world in recent decades. We often hear about the many successes it has in treating pain, but it has also proven itself to be extremely effective in helping treat a wide range of diseases. The World Health Organisation recognises the effectiveness of Acupuncture for more than sixty conditions from high blood pressure to infertility to the common cold, depression and anxiety, headaches, irritable bowel, the list goes on. Having that recognition helps but we as Acupuncturists know only too well, the amazing results we see daily and how peoples lives are changed on all levels when the body is brought back to balance. Acupuncture is not targeting the disease or pathogen; instead, it adjusts the function of the human body itself so that the body can heal. This "healing" is an innate ability we all have and as time goes by, I am constantly amazed by the resilience and strength we can all tap into with a little bit of help.

How Does Acupuncture Help?

Developed thousands of years ago, before the introduction of scientific research, the theory behind acupuncture is that Qi, or life force (or life energy), flows along pathways, also known as meridians, throughout the body. Disruption in these pathways can become problematic, causing short term or often chronic symptoms resulting in illness or disease. Along these pathways or meridians, we have approximately 365 acupuncture points that we commonly access, (not altogether of course!), by the insertion of fine needles, that can bring the energy flow or Qi, back into balance. The current studies of acupuncture suggest it can help with blood circulation, metabolism, gastrointestinal motility, heart rate, blood pressure, and immune function. It also produces endorphins, (natural pain killers), block pain signals going to the brain, has an anti-inflammatory effect and reduces the occurrence of muscle spasms. All of which, thanks to our advances in science and research, can now be visibly seen in a laboratory setting.

I will always remember my first ever encounter with an Acupuncturist, who it turned out I went on to train with for the next three years. She had a world of knowledge, gained from over twenty-five years in practice and experience. There was nothing she had not seen. She took my hand, invited me to sit down and without asking me any questions, she proceeded to tell me my body was burned out and that exhaustion and depletion had set in. My stomach was under duress and as a result, I was retaining fluid. I was possibly very hormonal, experiencing poor quality sleep, emotionally sad and frustrated and she could tell all this by just looking at my face, my tongue and taking a pulse check — which is not at all similar to the Western approach to checking our pulse. That was it. I was hooked! Everything she said was spot on and our conversation revolved around my confirming what I had been going through and my relevant symptoms. A plan was then put in place to help me get back to a place of balance and stability.

In Chinese philosophy, the principle of Yin and Yang is that all things exist as inseparable and contradictory opposites, for example, light–dark, young–old, black–white, hot–cold, day–night, and that these two opposites attract and complement each other and as their symbol illustrates, each side has at its core an element of the other (represented by the small dots). Neither pole is superior to the other and, as an increase in one brings a corresponding decrease in the other, a correct balance between the two poles must be reached to achieve harmony. And so, it is with our body, Yin representing the feminine, Yang representing the masculine, and we have qualities of each within us that together complete wholeness. When treating a person with Acupuncture, this balancing of Yin and Yang is at the centre of our objective whilst looking for patterns of excess or deficiency, internal or external, hot, or cold.

This holistic approach sees the 'person', body, mind, and spirit and encompasses all areas of their life to be gently recognised, held, explored and if necessary, healed. It cannot be about getting rid of a symptom quickly so one can get back on the daily grind of life to only re-create the pattern or problem again if there is no awareness brought to the original imbalance. There is a beautiful quote by Anais Nin: "We see the world not as it is, but as we are." and truly, that is how we perceive what is happening to us daily. Our belief systems can define what we experience as we see our lives played out through our trials, our dramas, our pain, our relationships, even our illness. However, if this is all happening unconscious to us, it may seem like we are a victim to our circumstances, but I believe it is quite the opposite. What if we drop the narrative around a situation, and through becoming more conscious, accept what is happening around us, embrace our discomfort, and see the power and strength we have to handle anything that comes our way?

It is not what happens to us that needs to be looked at, whether that be illness, shock, or trauma but our response to what has happened is much more important. We all experience things differently depending on our makeup and it is the greatest challenge of recovery to find who out we truly are in the midst of the pain and loss of control. The emotional and physical sensations become imprinted during these times and these continue to affect and disrupt not only our physiology but also our physical responses in the future. Acupuncture as a treatment has the precious ability to gently support the body, mental, physical, emotional, and spiritual while delving into the history of the story that is the physical ailment. Through a process of helping to calm the mind, we welcome awareness, then gently move what is stagnant or stuck in the muscles, tendons, ligaments, blood vessels, nerves, and energy centres of the body. It also helps support the deficient systems of the body, which have become exhausted through adrenal fatigue, burnout, stress, hormone imbalance or nutritional deficiency.

Fiona (not her real name), arrived to the clinic, a typical young professional, mid-thirties, high powered job, some late nights, lots of travel, never missed an early morning gym session and always following a schedule but never enough hours in the day. Her complaint was she lacked in energy, her periods were often late and always painful, her skin and hair had lost their lustre and she was having difficulty sleeping. However, she felt in complete 'control' of her life from a work perspective and as everything was on a schedule, she could not understand why at her age, she was feeling so weary. She just wanted her energy to return to how she used to feel in her early twenties. I listened to her carefully as she spoke and observed her dark circles under a beautifully made-up face, which could not hide the obvious signs of increasing fatigue. Her hair was tied up but indeed thin and lacklustre. She spoke like she was in a meeting at work, articulate and confident and you could see she wanted to feel like she had a finger on the pulse of what was happening, but in truth, she was agitated because this situation was outside of her control.

As we started to unwind her story, we began to tease out the energy vampires in her life — what drove her to early mornings, long days, restless nights, and an obvious lack of joy in her life? We discussed her lack of good nutrition, time out just for herself with nothing to do or nowhere to be, and she began to unravel as I gently teased out her relationship issues and in particular her history of growing up as the eldest child with a mom who suffered from crippling anxiety. In her early years, she took on the role of mothering her younger sister and brother and that required a lot of "control", everything needed to be on a schedule to ensure life ran smoothly while she tried to get through college and run a family home with military precision. There was no time for her feelings or needs, she was working day and night and it was routine for her to skip meals and ensure everybody else was looked after before herself.

This pattern had continued into her life today, even though she had long since left home, got married, moved away from the town where she was born but the programming, patterning and belief systems lived with her up to this moment, manifesting as her burnout, tired, stressed and emotionally drained body. Bringing her to this awareness was a key part of the road to recovery. She thought I was going to just try to 'fix' her energy levels and help her sleep better. I was going to do it as the therapist. Isn't that how it all works?

So, as with all my patients and for anybody who finds themselves sitting in my clinic, I am always at pains to stress that as a therapist, I will give them the very best of what I know and what I can do to HELP them help themselves and as a facilitator of that process, I hand them BACK the responsibility for their own healing. It is imperative to show everyone that they hold within themselves an innate ability to heal. What we have to do as a therapist in our particular field, is to bring awareness to the root cause of the situation first and sometimes that can be hard to face. To bring about change, we firstly must stop doing all the things we have been doing to see any potential difference, that is not so easy for some.

With Fiona, it took weeks of her seeing these patterns of "control" in her work and personal life, and to help her realise it was safe to let go and release the fear of doing so. That alone would have a physiological impact on her kidney energy. Therefore her adrenals could start to function better, her heart energy, which would impact her control issues, help calm her mind and initiate a better night's sleep. Once she acknowledged her emotional suppression, we decided a journal would be of huge benefit and she wrote down her feelings every day, regardless of how difficult she found it. Then the last thing at night, I got her to write down five things she was profoundly grateful for in that day just passed. As a result, her liver energy was able to move more freely, thus enabling less painful periods and a more relaxed body. Over time, she both laughed and cried, and the energy of her lungs could finally take a deep breath again, taking in all of life as it should be for her.

Small steps, simple changes, a recognition of where we can slowly turn things around that often seem impossible, and crucially, acceptance of where one is at right now are the key to letting a few small needles illicit such magnificent probabilities! Acupuncture is a different experience for everybody. I get asked quite often, do you have to believe in it for it to work, and my answer is always the same, just come with an open mind and together we focus our 'intention' on one thing, getting you better and letting the Acupuncture do what it does anyway!

Fiona and many like her are typical of what I get to see every day in my clinic. It may be that the emotional, nutritional, physical or spiritual symptoms appear at my door as Frank's migraine that is ever-present, Mary's irritable bowel that debilitates on a daily basis, John's constant neck and shoulder pain, Michelle's tennis elbow that persists despite injections, Aoife's autoimmune that is managed by pharmacological intervention — I could go on and on.

Unconsciously, we have committed our lives to be all things to all people, wearing a mask of what we think we should be to others so how we portray ourselves is blinded by the unconscious need for validation, acceptance, and approval. We have been conditioned from the moment we were conceived, and our lives remain a journey back to the greatest connection we have to healing, 'finding our own selves'. I hope in some small way that I have enlightened you to the beauty of the Acupuncture and Chinese medicine world and even more so, show you what is possible for your health and wellbeing once you are guided and nurtured along the way. You are never alone on this journey and whatever you believe, always know there is a higher power supporting and loving us unconditionally. Sometimes, we just need to get out of the way and allow our destiny to unfold as it will anyway!

Health does not always come from Medicine
Most of the time it comes from
peace of mind, peace in heart, peace of soul,
It comes from Laughter & Love

I can be contacted at www.galwayholistic.com.

Passion to Thrive
by Roberta Branagan

My name is Roberta. I have turned forty this year and have battled with my health since I was thirty, that is until I found Systematic Kinesiology and went on to train in it.

I have spent a lot of time in the medical system and had I known more about diet, nutrition and gut health and the importance of this, I might have a different story to tell.

I believed the story of "it runs in my family" around symptoms and illness. Now I say to people "bad food choices run in families".

I found Kinesiology because of my own poor health. Just before turning thirty, I started having pain in my arms and elbows. After getting bloods done with my GP, my CRP was raised, this is your C Reactive Protein and this measures inflammation in the body. I was referred to a rheumatologist and approximately a year later was diagnosed with fibromyalgia. During this time, I started on anti-inflammatory medication for pain, steroid injections into my elbows and anti-depressants for poor sleep. I had no knowledge or realisation of how much damage all these drugs were doing to my gut health, and I still felt awful most of the time. I often did not tell anyone how bad I was feeling physically inside of my body. It was hard to tell people as on the outside you look normal, but that is a long way from where your body is feeling on the inside.

Over time I was a zombie. I had two young children aged one and two and was working as a Senior Buyer in a medical device company which thankfully was mainly a desk job. I would come home from work and spend many evenings in bed with my boys watching cartoons on TV. I was not able to physically do anything else. This made me incredibly sad as a young mom of two boys that I was not able to run around after them. It made me angry. WHY ME? Why did this have to happen to me? What did I do wrong? Why can't I be like the other mums running around after their kids? I had no idea what Systematic Kinesiology was when I was told to visit one. I just had heard from a colleague that her sister had been to one for fibromyalgia. That was the start of my journey of love for Kinesiology.

Through this journey I dealt with a lot of emotional trauma that I had held onto for years — even since childhood. A lot of anger was causing pain in my shoulders. How is that even possible, I hear you say? I had held onto grief from the passing of my brother-in-law as during that time, I supported my husband and our kids over this loss and never grieved myself. This was also causing pain in my upper body as grief is held in the lung meridian as well as the large intestine meridian and I was prone to IBS too. I had grief from the loss of my grandparents, who I was incredibly close to.

Fibromyalgia is a disorder characterized by widespread musculoskeletal pain accompanied by fatigue, headache, depression, anxiety, memory, concentration, sleep and mood issues. Researchers believe that fibromyalgia amplifies painful sensations by affecting the way your brain processes pain signals.

This condition can be hard to understand, even for healthcare providers. Its symptoms mimic those of other conditions, and there are not any real tests to confirm the diagnosis. As a result, fibromyalgia is often misdiagnosed. Fibromyalgia causes what is now referred to as 'regions of pain.' Some of these regions overlap with what was previously referred to as areas of tenderness called 'trigger points' or 'tender points.'

Fibromyalgia symptoms have generally been more severe in women than in men. Women have more widespread pain, IBS symptoms, and morning fatigue than men. Painful periods are also common.

Some thoughts around what I have seen and in my opinion, fibromyalgia affects more women than men; those affected tend to come from a caring type role like nurses. A past illness could trigger fibromyalgia or make its symptoms worse. The flu, pneumonia, GI infections, such as those caused by Salmonella and Shigella bacteria, and the Epstein-Barr virus all have possible links to fibromyalgia.

Fibromyalgia often runs in families. If you have a family member with this condition, you are at higher risk of developing it. Researchers think certain gene mutations may play a role. They have identified a few possible genes that affect the transmission of chemical pain signals between nerve cells.

People who go through severe physical or emotional trauma may develop fibromyalgia. The condition has been linked to post -traumatic stress disorder (PTSD). Like trauma, stress can leave long-lasting effects on your body. Stress has been linked to hormonal changes that could contribute to fibromyalgia.

Over time I identified sleep and stress were my two triggers when it came to fibromyalgia. If either of those were not in the right proportion, I would ache all over. Alcohol and caffeine did not help either. I had to learn how to manage my stress more effectively to have a reasonable level of energy for work and family and then to sleep well, so the body healed nightly. There were days at work in the canteen when my hands could not even carry the tray of lunch; they were trembling with weakness.

There are times I still find it hard to peel potatoes with my hands aching from the repetitive action.

From early outset, I was determined not to be defined by fibromyalgia; it was not me and I was not it. I went back to college to complete my degree at thirty-two and it was an immensely proud moment graduating from Trinity with my Business Degree having my kids with me to celebrate. At thirty-five, I decided I was going to walk the Camino de Santiago (a bucket list item) and I was certainly not going to let fibro stop me either. One hundred kilometres later, I had earned my certificate and had lots of 'ah-ha!' moments throughout.

I had changed jobs and went into a start-up type business in Supply Chain and things just plummeted from there. The stress was enormous. The job was all-consuming and my diet went downhill. I used sugar to cope and to keep going on the hamster wheel. I used wine to help me fall asleep at night and then diet drinks the next day to keep me going, along with lots of caffeine.

It was around this time that I had been going to a Kinesiologist and my thyroid kept showing up as imbalanced during muscle testing. A high percentage of fibromyalgia patients will have a thyroid disorder, something like thirty-three percent. I had to beg to get to see an endocrinologist. My bloods with regards to my TSH (Thyroid Stimulating Hormone) were on the rise but not within the range to be an issue. I had all the other symptoms, fatigue, rough, dry skin, deepened voice, excess weight gain around the mid-section. Even when my bloods fell within the range FINALLY, I was like "Yes I'll get sorted now." Then my GP said, "Oh sure we will wait another six months and re-do bloods." I was almost broken. I don't know how I found the inner strength to sit in their office and say that if you do not refer me to an endocrinologist I will go and sit in A&E until someone can help me. The letter she wrote to refer me was unbelievable, making out I was unstable.

I remember being on more than one family holiday and having to pull out the work laptop to go online and do some month-end reports or similar. It was ridiculous. Amid this stressful work environment, I had challenging relationships going on with family living with us as well as immediate family on both sides. It was too much for my mind and I ended up crying in my new GP's office after going through a few very scary panic attacks and knew that this was anxiety and I could not deal with it myself. I realised I had anxiety since childhood but never knew that this was the word to describe this feeling.

My new GP was incredible. I was adamant initially that I was not going on medication and I started some sessions in counselling which left me exhausted and emotional every Thursday and each weekend for several weeks. I was drained. I felt it was me that was the common denominator and it had to be all my fault. Since training in other modalities, I realised that there is a responsibility on both parties. I have handed back all responsibilities that were not mine to the other parties. Another Kinesiologist said to my kids once, if your brother invites you to row or fight do you have to accept? I went back to my GP and started a course of medication for anxiety and that helped me as a short-term gap that I needed to deal with all of life that was happening at that time.

Thankfully, I was made redundant from my job and had some finance to invest in training courses while looking for a job. This was me starting my journey with health and wellbeing. I started with IET and Reiki. Then some weeks later I spotted a basics course in Systematic Kinesiology called Balanced Health. I decided to do this to use the knowledge for myself and my family until I was hooked and doing a Diploma in Systematic Kinesiology and then setting up a clinic and leaving the job I had started in Project Management.

I had started the new job around the same time I started the Kinesiology course. Of course over time this job became stressful working long hours and days and work flowing into my family life and me being irritable because I was stressed. I was the only one that couldn't see I was stressed.

The Kinesiology training took place over two years and I finally felt I had found my tribe. These people got me, and they knew how I felt. They too had their own reasons for doing the training. They too had their own traumas and crap that life had thrown at them.

During each weekend of training, I cried, and I cried, and I cried some more. I had no idea where all these tears had been stored. The tears were for a whole range of different issues. We use a technique called Past Trauma Recall and this can use muscle testing to pinpoint an age at which something traumatic occurred and figure out how to help the body's muscle memory clear it. I like to tell clients it is the opposite to a memory foam mattress; the muscle does not bounce back it stays with the imprint in it until you deal with the trauma and it allows the body to heal.

During this time, I started to feel better or as people working in holistic therapies will call it 'heal'.

It was freeing. We used techniques for affirmations around loving yourself. I did not realise that my body did not feel loved; how awful is that? It reverted back to age fourteen, and using a technique called Eye Rotations, "I released the feelings of being unloved" while then using another technique called Temporal Tapping to establish "I am loved with all my faults and failings", while muscle testing to see which Bach Remedy would help clear those feelings.

I spent so much time feeling like I was not good enough that I had to retrain my brain and my body that I was more than good enough, that I loved myself. Every training weekend, I was blown away with the secrets muscle testing was revealing as well as learning so many techniques involved in helping the body recover.

Unfortunately, during this time, as much as my emotional health started to improve my physical health was on a very slippery slope. I felt extremely hot one day in work and asked the onsite health person could I get my temperature checked. She checked my blood pressure which was sky-high. This was the warning sign my body was giving me to STOP. Up to this point, I took each stressful situation on the chin and kept going. My body had a different idea. I was not listening to the warning signs I was too busy.

Soon after I was diagnosed with high blood pressure and had to go on medication, I was thirty-seven. From here, other things started developing. My thyroid consultant did a questionnaire assessment with me and sent me to a sleep apnoea specialist for review. I had to wear a machine with wires everywhere for my sleep assessment, and I was diagnosed with obstructive sleep apnoea.

Lack of quality sleep was causing major fatigue all day long and of course, add in stress and my body was ready to explode. I now had three consultants at thirty-seven. This was not a good sign. Again, this is not how I wanted to be defined. I went on a CPAP machine, which is horrendous to get used to and kids and hubby started called me Darth Vader.

During the second year of training, we had a weekend on Leaky Gut. This made so much sense and was really where the physical healing of my body started. I had every pathogen that was in the kit. With Systematic Kinesiology, we work with priority in the body, which area does the body want to work on first? The healing of my gut started with my mercury fillings. I made the decision to get them removed with full approval from my dentist.

I had done so much research around fibromyalgia and had seen some around mercury, so for me it made sense when it showed up in muscle testing.

I discovered that I had a lactose intolerance as well as a gluten intolerance which was irritating my gut each time, I consumed them. This explained a lot of the IBS feelings of bloating, constipated and then diarrhoea. I found it difficult to remove gluten from my diet more than the lactose in dairy.

Muscle testing showed parasites, fungus, and virus EBV in my gut, and slowly but surely with a priority of what the body wanted to work on. I was on my way to healing my gut. I started drinking fresh celery juice in the mornings. When I started it was horrible, which is an indication of toxins in the body. Vitamins, supplements, and minerals all aided in my gut healing as well.

I started sleeping better, eating better, more energy, I started regaining my life, I was able to stop using my CPAP as I had started losing weight there was less pressure on the soft tissue in the neck. My blood pressure regulated itself and I was able to slowly wean off the medication with my GP's support. I had already weaned myself off the anxiety medication as well and was feeling happier in myself and more content.

I had gone from taking anti-inflammatory, anti-depressants, steroid injections, blood pressure medication, anxiety medication, CPAP machine, thyroid medication to celery juice.

It has been a rollercoaster ride which I know is a cliché. I have now come to the conclusion that my own journey of self -discovery and healing is one to be proud of. Had I not had adversity then it would be harder for me to empathise and help my own clients that come and trust me with their wellbeing.

I look at the hardship as the reason I changed and the reason for where I am now with my 'job' as a Kinesiologist and I am grateful for those hard times and the change. If I had continued the stressed path I was on, I would have had more and more health challenges coming my way.

Kin–easy–ology

I could not pronounce it when I first went for a session and during training one of the other practitioners spelt it out this way, brilliant, people are less afraid of it when they can say it.

I was asked once by a parent who is a teacher to describe in one sentence what Kinesiology does?

Systematic Kinesiology uses muscle testing to find imbalances in the body. This will identify the source of health issues, whether its nutritional, emotional, structural, or mental. Then we get into the nitty-gritty as they say and start clearing out what the body is holding onto.

There are forty-two muscles that we work with in the body and fifteen meridians, each muscle relates to one of the meridians. Often in the medical world, we have a view of looking at everything individually and do not see the connection with the whole body.

A pain in the back can be a structural problem if pulled or twisted and equally it can be caused by the emotional trauma of not feeling supported. Sore knees could be from the weight of a broken heart. A thyroid problem could be from holding in all the things you want to say and cannot, causing an energy blockage of your throat chakra.

I have heard something about it, but I am not sure what it is — sound familiar?

Kinesiology can help with more than eighty percent of all health problems that most people put up with, either because it is not bad enough to go for medical treatment or they have already sought help but received no relief. Just feeling below par or a bit under the weather seems to be the norm. It is accepted as a normal way of life. It does not have to be that way.

Systematic Kinesiology treats the whole person — mind, body, biochemistry, and energy. Treating imbalances in the body by resolving a problem in one area, will leave a positive effect throughout the whole body, as everything in the body is connected.

What Happens In A Session?

The client is fully clothed on the plinth and asked to move their arms and legs in different positions to test a specific muscle. The kinesiologist places gentle pressure against the arm or leg for two or three seconds. If the muscle is working properly, it will stay firm and steady. If there is an imbalance, the arm or leg will move under this pressure or feel spongy to the kinesiologist. This gives us the start of a clue of what is going on in the client's body.

Next, we start looking at identifying why the muscle is not working correctly and if it is a compensation imbalance (not the real problem) or the cause of the imbalance. We break this down into what we call MCPE – Mental, Chemical, Physical and Energetic to determine the root cause of the muscle not working. I aim to explain this further below so you can understand how this works.

Mentally

Mental balance in the body is considered as a cheerful and optimistic outlook. Mental balance can help restore balance to the brain's ability to think positivity and effectively to relieve emotional stress quicker. Other views would be the absence of anxiety and freedom of fear. If you asked most people, they have some fear or other. Some are known fears like the fear of a dog as they had been bitten as a child or an unknown fear like of flying and no reason for it. People's fear ranges from spiders, dogs, or other animals to fear of the dark, open spaces. Flying is a common one which prevents people from travelling, and even fear of dying. My own biggest one was fear of failure, particularly leaving a pensioned job to move into being self-employed. People felt they could even say to me "Are you crazy leaving a pensioned job?"

Lack of sleep can leave us mentally drained, so it is important to get a good night's sleep, complete rest, and relaxation. There are many reasons why people do not get enough sleep at night. Exercise daily is difficult if we are always rushing and chasing the clock with work, dropping and collecting kids from school or sports, little time left for yourself to exercise. Even thirty minutes a day for a walk is supporting your mental health and helping the body stay in balance.

Water plays so many important roles in the body, yet we take it for granted and do not drink enough. Can it really be that simple, a headache caused by lack of water? Every organ needs water to work especially the brain, so when it does not have enough the body gets tight, muscles get tight which in turn affects the joints, bones, etc. and our body does not function correctly and gives you signals. For example a headache often ignored or a pain killer taken, whereas water in some cases could solve the problem, little and often, throughout the day so the body can absorb it. Lots of techniques that can be used to support the mental realm of the body like Fundamental Conflicts, Temporal Tapping, Emotional Stress Release (ESR), Past Trauma Recall and Bach Flower Remedies in isolation or combined.

The Bach Flower Remedies is a system of thirty-eight Flower Remedies discovered by Dr Edward Bach more than eighty years ago. The Bach Flower Remedies remove negative emotions by flooding them with positive energies from flowers. I personally love these for myself, my family and they work wonders with clients, often shifting stuck negative energies and thoughts.

Physically

Physically we work on the lymphatic points on the body. Lymphatic fluid needs the body to move the muscles for it to pump around the body, unlike blood which is pumped by the heart around the body. Lymphatic fluid needs movement and due to the lifestyle most of us lead, we don't get lymph moving as freely as it should. We sit in the car to and from work, sitting in the office at a desk and sitting in the evening, so it's quite easy for fluid to get stuck. By walking at a minimum every day will encourage the lymph to continue to move, or any exercise which creates movement within the body.

I will often give clients 'homework' and it could be to massage these lymphatic points at home post-appointment and it will help keep their symptoms at bay for slightly longer by following this advice.

We need to work towards good posture, strong structure and balanced muscles. Sometimes if the left side of the neck isn't working correctly this is considered a weakened muscle. The pain of that is often felt on the right side as the muscle there is taking up the slack of the weakened muscle. Clients are often fascinated that I work on the muscle opposite to where the pain is. Or even a pain on the left side of the neck could cause a problem with the right hip as the muscles stack.

We have a range of cranial techniques that are beneficial as part of the physical realm. We muscle test the cranial technique against the client's body to see if they need this adjustment.

Chemically

Chemically or nutritionally the muscle could need a vitamin or supplement for it to work to its full potential, often we do not eat a balanced diet that gives us everything we need to support our body. Most people do not eat even green leafy vegetables, therefore are lacking magnesium. This could show as constipation in the client or restless legs or even anxiety or sleep issues. Magnesium promotes healthy muscles helping them relax and especially great for PMS. It is important for the nervous system and aids restful sleep as well as being essential for energy production – involved as a cofactor in over three hundred functions in the body.

Stress can cause havoc with the body and will use up a lot of our Vitamin C, so during stressful times, I always advise clients to increase their intake of Vitamin C using supplementation. Vitamin C strengthens the immune system and supports the adrenals. Deficiency of Vitamin C will show up as frequent colds or infections, lack of energy and easy bruising.

On the flip side, we could be eating food or drinking fizzy drinks or alcohol that switches off our muscles from performing. The main culprits are gluten and dairy along with caffeine and sugar.

I get little babies who are formula-fed having all sorts of problems like reflux, vomiting, waking at night, chronic diarrhoea, or constipation and as soon as we switch to goats or soya formula, the baby is like a different little person. Same goes for kids and adults.

We all have a toxic load and depending on our lifestyle, we can reach that limit which can cause chronic digestive issues that we never even link together. Think about what you use on your body from when you wake to when you sleep, the products you use in the shower. Post shower you use antiperspirants, perfumes, aftershaves, and for many ladies a whole range of cosmetics. These are all full of different chemicals and to one man it is no issue, but to another whose reaching their toxic load, it can be the last straw for the body. Then you throw in a couple of coffees, some fizzy drinks, gluten, dairy and a bucket load of stress and you can really understand how the body is struggling.

We use test kits to check the client's body using muscle testing for a reaction to the vials to see if the client has an intolerance to certain food types. We recommend the client makes a list of foods they consume in an average week and ask them to bring some of them with them to the appointment especially if they are specific brands or types that the client uses.

Energetically

Balancing the meridians within the body will leave the body feeling more energised. We use a couple of things to help balance energies.

I personally love working with chakras. There are seven of them — Root, Sacral, Solar Plexus, Heart, Throat, Third Eye and Crown. Chakras are an energy field that we cannot see and extend out about three inches from the body. Each one relates to a certain area in the body, certain colours, (colours of the rainbow) and even certain musical notes and can cause a physical or emotional imbalance in the body.

We might need to look at avoiding stressful people who drain our energies, and you will know who they are. Electronic stress, like excessively phone usage and blue light, are to be avoided.

Can It Help Me? Can It Help A Loved One?

Kinesiology helps with a whole range of issues, from emotional to nutritional to back pain. It is suitable for all ages, and all mobility ranges.

We have an incredibly unique technique called surrogate testing that we can use another person to surrogate test to get feedback, so for little babies to older people, kinesiology can help with all ages.

My youngest client was eight weeks and my oldest was eighty-three so far!

Kinesiology can help with so many imbalances in the body. I will name the most common areas that people with seek help from a Kinesiologist.

- Muscular aches and pains
- Hormonal and fertility imbalances
- Depression and anxiety
- Stress release and management
- Fears and phobias
- Physical and emotional trauma
- Food intolerances, gut, and digestive issues
- Sleep
- Fatigue
- Confidence and self-esteem

My own specialist areas would be working with children around sleep and anxiety and because of my own health journey, I do a lot of work around Fibromyalgia, Thyroid and Gut Health.

The reference sources I quoted from are *An Introduction to Kinesiology and Kinesiology for Balanced Health*, both by Brian Butler.

Testimonials

Hi Roberta, well done on writing the book. It is excellent to get awareness out there for Kinesiology.

I was diagnosed with fibromyalgia in 2017. I did not know much about it at the time and did not know how to deal with my symptoms. My sister had spotted a video on Facebook of a lady who had fibromyalgia and practiced kinesiology, which helps fibromyalgia symptoms. As it happens, I had met Roberta before through my husband.

I was under a lot of stress at work which made my symptoms worse. I could not cope with the pain and tiredness. Roberta was doing a study on people with fibromyalgia and how it helped. I joined the study and have not looked back.

My first appointment was strange as I did not know anything about Kinesiology. Roberta put me at ease then gave me a form to point out my symptoms and areas of pain. Straight away, Roberta gave me some tips to help symptoms. Like taking Vitamin C and magnesium. I was then muscle tested and I was amazed that muscle test pointed out areas of pain and whether they were emotional or structural.

The difference between the first and second appointment was like chalk and cheese. The reduction in my symptoms was big. As the appointments went on, Roberta helped me more with my diet, vitamin supplements, affirmations, as well as my pain which was greatly reduced.

I go back to Roberta for top-up appointments when I get a flare-up of symptoms. I cannot recommend Roberta or kinesiology enough. I even brought my nine-year-old daughter, who suffers from anxiety to Roberta. Thanks – **Toni.**

Initially I brought my twelve-year-old son to see Roberta as he was feeling tired and had no energy, which was not like him at all! I had brought him to the doctor they could not see anything wrong, but he still was not right!!

I had never heard of Kinesiology before, but I was on Facebook one night and I came across RB Holistic I made an appointment we went to Roberta not really knowing what to expect but after our session and within a couple of days, he was starting to come back to himself we could all see the change in him, even our neighbours noticed the change in him!!

I decided to bring my other son who was fourteen to Roberta next as he lacked in concentration and no energy and not sleeping very well, after his session he said he had the best sleep he had in ages and we noticed a complete change in him. He had an interest in things, his energy improved and he was even getting up on time for school!!!

I said I would make an appointment for myself. I have high blood pressure, an underactive thyroid, I did not realise I felt so bad until I started feeling good after my sessions with Roberta!!

My body was stressed to the last. I had aches and pains thinking I had injuries, but it was stress. Roberta worked on me. I had to have a few sessions and it is the most relaxing and balancing treatment I have ever experienced. I have never felt better, and as I said, I didn't realise I felt so bad until I started feeling good!

I made an appointment for my husband who has rheumatoid arthritis. The first day he went he could hardly lie on the bed in Roberta's clinic, his back was so sore. He had so much stress in his body as well, but after a few sessions with Roberta he has never felt better, his mood, his energy, his body, he is even able to do exercise now and enjoy it which he never could before.

We all had great sleep the night after our sessions and within a few days, started feeling better myself, and my husband are in our forties and I can honestly say we have never felt better, we have gone back even though we didn't really need to, but I feel it is a treat to ourselves to have a kinesiology session now!

Kinesiology is gentle, non-invasive, and totally relaxing. I cannot recommend it highly enough!!

I have told my friends, work colleagues, everyone about kinesiology because it really has made a difference in our lives for the whole family. Kind regards – **Siobhan.**

So how am I now? I will have turned forty, happy that I changed my life for the better and not just my own but my familys'. They are growing up with a happier mom, who is less critical of herself and is giving them a good understanding and grounding for what health is about both mentally and physically. We openly talk about our emotions, the good days and the bad.

I still have the odd bad day and roll with that. I currently do not take medication for blood pressure, blood sugar, thyroid, fibromyalgia, or anxiety and glad to say the CPAP machine has been packed away forever. I do take supplements like the ones mentioned in the chapter: predominantly magnesium, selenium, zinc, Vitamin D and C as I know that they are what is needed for my body. I juice celery two to three times a week, and I drink three litres of water daily. I meditate when I can or feel the need to. I love Pilates, and with lockdown, I started playing golf with my boys.

I'm losing weight slowly but surely only after I have done all the work I have as mentioned in this chapter – this is what I tell clients all the time. Weight is a symptom and often not the problem like we think it is. I was always obsessed about my weight and judged my happiness on being skinnier until I was and realised that it really had nothing to do with it.

My stress levels are well below normal, and I plan to keep them there. I love that my job as a Kinesiologist not just helps my family and me but others too. A lot of my clients tend to be clusters of a family and they all love how Kinesiology makes them feel and that gives me great joy, particularly working with children and giving them tools for their lives.

I have met so many fabulous therapists throughout, and we meet up and share our therapies with each other and it is a great way to maintain self-care in a job where we care for everyone that comes through our doors.

Little Tips And Tricks That May Help You

- **Look at what you are putting into your body, both food and chemicals**

  Keep a food diary and notice things like sugar, gluten, dairy, alcohol and even your water intake, and things like what fruit or vegetables you consume each day/week.

  Look at making sure you are getting the correct nutritional support, and getting the following key nutrients either from your food or supplementation

  As well as already mentioning Vitamin C and Magnesium throughout the chapter, these four are the other regular ones that show for clients in muscle testing.

- **Vitamin D Deficiency**

  Joint pain or stiffness, backache, tooth decay, muscle cramps, hair loss, low mood

- **Zinc Deficiency**

  Poor sense of taste or smell, frequent infections, stretch marks, acne or greasy skin, low fertility, pale skin, a tendency to depression, loss of appetite

- **Selenium Deficiency**

  Signs of premature ageing, high blood pressure, frequent infections, healthy thyroid

- **Probiotics Deficiency**

  Diarrhoea, Candida, Digestive disorders, low immune system slow to recover from illness allergies, eczema, asthma, dermatitis

- **Adrenal Stress – Points to rub when stressed**
  Find your belly button, measure one inch out and two inches up from there, either side, massaging these points at the end of the day to release stress from the body is so beneficial at helping the body. These points are the neuro lymphatic points for the Adrenals.

- **ESR – Emotional Stress Release**
  Just some of the benefits of ESR technique is emotional balance, relief from tension and helping with overwhelm. If you think about it, a lot of us do this automatically when we hear bad news. We tend to put our hand to our forehead. It's the body's natural way of soothing itself. In the clinic, I incorporate ESR with past trauma, current stress and future ESR maybe for exam nerves or interview nerves, with Bach remedies, DoTerra oils, vitamin or mineral support, guided by what the body needs.

- **Bach Flower Remedies**
  In the clinic, I incorporate several techniques like ESR or Fundamental Conflicts with the Bach Remedies to further give relief and balance to clients. I have listed the six most used remedies in the clinic that may resonate with you.
  - Walnut – changes in life, college, exams, job, wedding, house
  - Elm – overwhelmed with responsibilities
  - Olive – racing mind–helps with sleep
  - Aspen/Mimulus – Unknown/Known Fears
  - Holly – Anger

- **Temporal Tapping** is a way of reprogramming how you want to be.

  I generally tell clients to stick to the left side and positive statement, for example – I will eat healthily – I make good choices around food. The subconscious does not know the difference between real and unreal and temporal tapping bypasses the logic filter.

- **Thymus Tapping**

  This is a simple but amazing technique where you tap the thymus. It is in the upper part of the chest directly behind your sternum and between your lungs. The thymus is part of the endocrine system. As we get older past puberty, it starts getting smaller. This is like a jump start to the immune system. This tapping needs to be done to the rhythm of waltz music. This is linked to self-esteem and human love, so I often get clients to tap and use affirmations like 'I love myself', or 'I love myself with all my faults and failings'.

- **Cross Crawl**

  This is an exercise to stimulate the brain. It is marching on the spot, crossing your left arm over to touch your right knee and vice versa. Do this regularly, especially to some of your favourite music to make it more fun. This will help stimulate the flow of vital Cerebral-Spinal Fluid and yields great benefits, including balance emotions, blood pressure, co-ordination, digestion, improving memory and even helps reduce stress.

To find out more, check out my website, Instagram, Facebook pages under RB Holistic Therapies.
https://www.rbholistictherapies.ie/

Breathing Life Into Me
by Suzanne Clarke

Imagine thinking that stress was a normal way to feel ALL the time? I did for an awfully long time and did not even realise it. My name is Suzanne Clarke and I am a Leadership & Wellbeing Coach and Yoga teacher living in Oranmore, Co. Galway. I am originally from Cork and moved to Galway over twenty years ago, after some time in London and abroad and I fell in love with the place. I met my husband David, working for the same company and we had our beautiful family.

Our jobs were busy with both of us away a lot, meaning constant juggling and organising the children, which was hard work. We relied on crèches, neighbours, friends, and our amazing families who were as supportive as they could be, even though they lived miles away from us. I felt asking for more help meant I was not able to manage things and I was always the strong, independent one, so I should still do it all. I thought being busy all the time was a good thing. Everyone else around me was busy too and they seemed to be making it work, I could too. Any of that sound familiar?

Writing this brings me straight back to how I felt at that time and how physically and mentally drained I was. I was a bit of a people pleaser, a bit of a perfectionist and afraid to say I could not do it all. I was great at pretending everything was alright, had no boundaries and no idea what they even meant and was afraid of letting go of control in case all the plates came crashing down. They had come crashing down a few years previously, when I miscarried my second baby, my little girl Lucy. My son was six-months-old when I found out I was pregnant, and David and I were both shocked and delighted at being pregnant again so soon.

I remember waking up at 5 am that morning in searing pain, driving into the hospital on the phone to my GP, knowing deep down what was happening. I remember thinking that maybe I was having twins and that maybe one would survive, trying to find some comfort in the reality of what was really going on. I knew in my heart what was happening, but my mind was trying to come up with as many solutions — anything but the truth. It was just not meant to be though. In the end, it was just me and Lucy in the hospital together and although she made it into the world briefly, it left me very traumatised. I did get a chance to say goodbye and can now see this now as a huge blessing, so many mums do not ever get that chance. I took a few days off work and went straight back into full-on work mode again, believing that was the best way to deal with it all. Everyone gave me that advice, so I thought that is what I had to do.

One thing I have learned from my own experience is that I will never ever offer that advice to anyone who has experienced this loss. I buried these feelings and did not properly mourn her, but like any emotion, we do not face, it came up years later in a different form. I was filled with guilt, blamed myself, was it my fault, did I want her enough, how would I cope with two small babies, how would I do my job, be mum, be a wife and keep it all going? Grief is a long, hard road. You think you have cried all your tears and there are none left, but then something is said, or a memory will trigger you and bring you right back to that time again. I have learned it is a process you have to go through, and you need support all along the way.

Not long after that, I got news one Christmas of a school friend of mine who had suffered a severe stroke, completely out of the blue. *This is what changed everything for me.* With the way I was living, always running and racing, I knew something else was going to happen involving my health, my marriage, something, and I just was not going to let that happen. It was a big wake up call for me of how I was going through the motions and not actually living. I left my 'secure' job and put myself out in the world as a yoga teacher. I can still remember putting my first flyer through the door, my fingers inside the letterbox and knowing I had to let go. Talk about feeling the fear and doing it anyway!

I can honestly say, yoga has totally transformed my life, is part of who I am and what I do now. So how did I get here?

Like a lot of people, I signed up to my first yoga class because of physical pain in my body. My lower back was causing me so much pain after years of long hours of driving in my job. A friend of mine, who was fed up listening to me complaining about it, invited me to come to a class he had just signed up for. I went along, not knowing what to fully expect. I had attended a class or two in my early twenties, but at that time, it just was not for me.

I remember feeling nervous going into that class. Everyone looked relaxed, some lying down, some stretching and looked like they knew what they were doing. The teacher started with a grounding practice which was totally alien to me and the class began moving from one pose to the other. My body was stiff in places I never knew existed and some of the postures I did not do because I just was not able to! The one pose I loved was a downward-facing dog, but after two or three, I was exhausted! After finishing the hour class, I was completely exhausted but exhilarated at the same time. I slept like a baby that night.

The next day, I woke up feeling every bit of the after-effects of the class, but it felt different to a normal gym workout or exercise class. I went back for more and before long, I was going twice a week. My lower back had never felt so good! I found my yoga class the best cure for a one-day return Galway–Donegal drive, better than anything else I had done before and believe me, I had tried everything.

After about two months of practicing twice a week, I found myself getting stronger. I looked forward to my downward dogs and started to enjoy them. My balance and focus improved and I was feeling great ease in my body. One evening, I was at class and not sure why, but I noticed how my teacher always spoke about the breath in his instruction during class.

"What is he talking about, sure don't we all breathe?" Honestly, they were my exact thoughts at the time, and he kept repeating this week after week. It was like an irritating itch that would not go away until I scratched it. As we set our intentions at the start of class, I decided to make mine listen to his prompts on breathing and try to understand just what he was talking about.

What happened after that was the start of my journey to becoming a yoga teacher. For the first time ever, I felt my breath and became conscious of HOW I was breathing. My practice felt different but still did not understand why. At the end of the class lying on the floor in relaxation, I felt a surge of emotion throughout my body, heard a voice inside me and tears came pouring out of me. And yes, I was mortified! My teacher did not blink an eye, though, as if it were the most normal thing in the world. I am eternally grateful for that, knowing now that it is so normal and that most of us do not ever allow ourselves to release emotion freely, not to mention in a public class. I left that class with big red eyes but felt amazing! What the hell had just happened, what were those feelings and who was that voice inside me screaming to be heard? Of course, I now know that it was me. I had let my body get so stressed, physically, mentally, and emotionally with how I was living, and I had gotten so used to it, I did not know any other way to be. This was not how my life used to be.

After finishing school, all I wanted to do was travel. The poor Presentation Sisters did not know what to do with me when it came to career guidance. "I just want to travel, Sister." was my line after every session. There was an overwhelming feeling inside me that I had to travel and see the world; it was all I wanted to do. My parents were so supportive when I told them and with one small suitcase and a duvet under my arm, I left home at nineteen after training as a beauty and massage therapist and headed to London. I slept on my friend's floor for a couple of weeks until I got my own place. I loved the buzz of London so much and worked right in the heart of it all. It was so exciting! I met people from all walks of life, all nationalities, so different from my life in Cork. I worked for Virgin Atlantic Airways for a while too, got to meet incredible people and my need for travel continued. Eventually, I came home to Ireland and back to Cork. My travelling bug was not over, and I moved to Galway, not knowing anyone and got a job with a pharmaceutical company. I was out and about meeting consultants, nurses, and patients all day in hospitals and doing something I really enjoyed. As the years went on, the job was becoming more demanding,all the driving was taking its toll on my body and I ignored it.

Discovering my breath at that yoga class, I knew I had to find out more. This is what led me to my teacher-training course to understand more about this experience, but I never intended to teach. The course was truly life-changing. It was physically and mentally challenging and had me in tears (again) a few times! I discovered a part of me that I had shut off and it had finally found its voice. I trained here in Ireland over thirteen months with the help of some truly incredible teachers. I met such an amazing bunch of people during my training, all with their own stories and reasons for being there and I learned so much from them. One weekend, I decided to clean out my garage and set it up as my Yoga Room where I taught my classes.

Through my own yoga practice, I have become so much more aware of my body and mind in such a way that now I know the signs, whether I am stressed, worried, need time away or just feeling off. I never had this ability before and looking back, I know I lost a huge piece of myself for a while trying to keep everything going. I realise throughout my life I had made intuitive choices in every decision I had ever made. If it *felt* right, then I went with it. Yoga has heightened this, even more, when it comes to my own needs and now those of others, which I did not expect. I am learning to trust my intuition/gut feeling again like I used to more and more. As a teacher, I am aware of the energy of my students now, too when they come into my class and vary my classes accordingly.

The joy I get from teaching yoga is watching people change from when they come to class, and when they are leaving class. New students will be nervous, shy, suspicious, and holding their body in a very protective way — just like I was in my first class. My job is to make sure they feel comfortable with me, with the group, the space and with their newfound practice. Regular students may know what to expect when they come to class, but still have problems and challenges they are dealing with. It is my job whatever the stage of the student, to be fully present and in tune with each one to the best of my ability. Sometimes that is challenging for me, but my intention is always to show up and do my best. Encouraging each student to stay with yoga during the tough times is one of my goals as a teacher. Sometimes as with everything you start in life and as our lives are so busy, you want to feel better straight away, and if you feel no benefit, perhaps frustration sets in, other things become more important and you give up.

Yoga is a process you go through requiring a commitment to yourself, consistency, patience and trusting what comes up for you. There are days after all these years that I just do not want to get on my mat, but I am never disappointed when I do. Watching someone change physically, mentally, emotionally in one hour is beautiful and I am so honoured to witness it and hold the space for them. Seeing this change in people and conversations after class with my students, I felt I wanted to do more for them. People left my class so differently but headed straight back into their stressful lives again. This led me on to the work I do now.

As a Leadership and Wellbeing coach, I help people to make further changes, discover their inner leadership, manage their stress, their overwhelm and enhance their wellbeing. Coaching is such a magical safe space for people to look at themselves, how they are living, their values, beliefs and make small changes that can have long – lasting effects. Yoga is that same magical space that does the same thing in a different way, but both complement each other perfectly. This is my work now, using both yoga and coaching to help women, young adults and teenagers manage their stress and overwhelm, find the joy and confidence in their lives and I love it!

A Brief History Of Yoga

Yoga has been around for over five thousand years and a practice and philosophy that originated in India. It takes its name from a classical language called Sanskrit which means "to unite or join together" and was originally practiced by men only. I believe yoga is really a way of living. Its aim is to bring body, mind and spirit into harmony using postures, breathe control and meditation to do this. Like anything else, being consistent with your practice, you get stronger, more flexible, have improved mobility, and maintain good health. Yoga helps you process your thoughts and emotions, allowing you to respond instead of reacting and make better choices, especially when things in life become challenging.

Yoga was introduced to the West in the 1900s by Indian monks, but it wasn't until the 1950s and 1960's that it became popular. Even though it was originally designed for men, women make up over eighty percent of an average class now and in some of my classes, it is more like one hundred percent.

In my own history of yoga, it is simply one of the best tools I know to feel better. It is something you can do anywhere, anytime and practicing it on days when you are tired, fed up or on the "just don't want to do anything" days will always make you feel better. It is a moving connection you make with yourself on every level, physical, emotional, mental, and spiritual. It meets you where you are and how you are feeling every time you get on the mat and it is suitable for EVERY single body of every age.

So What Is Yoga?

When you think of yoga, what comes into your head? Maybe you imagine a person sitting cross-legged or standing on one leg. Maybe you think of someone chanting or upside down in a headstand. Maybe it is more like an exercise class where you sweat and work hard. You are right!

Yoga can be all those things and yet it is so much more.

The framework or guidelines for this practice are called the Eight Limbs of Yoga. A book called *The Sutras of Patanjali* describes the eight limbs and this book is recommended to anyone looking to deepen their practice or simply learn more about the mind and meditation. I would like to offer my understanding of the eight limbs as simply as I can and how they are co-dependant on each other, one not being more important than the other. All the names are in Sanskrit and I hope I do justice to them all when offering my understanding.

Yama's

These are ethical rules or ways of living and there are five of them. They focus on the relationship we have with ourselves and the world around us

Ahimsa – Non-violence. This means causing no harm to others and to ourselves, not just physically, but emotionally too. How do you speak to others? How do you speak to yourself? How can you be aware of your actions and be kind to others today? How can you be kind to yourself today?

Satya – this means truth the word SAT means 'true essence.' It encourages us to think, speak and act with integrity, seeing things as they are and not how we wish them to be. As we all see things from our own perspective and from experiences we may have had, this can be different for everyone.

Asteya – Non stealing. As with all the other Yama's, this goes further than stealing an object from someone. How do you steal from yourself? Do you believe in yourself; do you have feelings of not being good enough, not having enough? Do you steal people's time?

Brahmacharya – using your energy right. This is about directing your energy away from external desires and finding peace and contentment within yourself. Moderation in everything as my grandad used to say!

Aparigraha – Non greed. This Yama encourages you to take only what you need in everything you do, hold on to only what serves you and let go when time is right.

As you will see, one Yama is linked to the next. When you are not kind to yourself, it may lead to dishonesty, greediness, and feelings of not having enough – same thing when you are on the mat. Being unkind to yourself, you may force yourself into shapes you are not ready for, causing stress on the body, frustration with yourself and the practice and feelings of not being good enough

– these simple, yet not so simple ways of living weave in and out of one another.

Niyama's

Attitudes and ways of being to cultivate in ourselves. Just like the yamas, there are five of them too.

Shaucha – Purity of the body and mind, both external and internal. You take a shower every day to remove impurities and keep you fresh, how often do you clean your internal body? What you eat, drink, the information you consume, how you move and what you think is all part of this Niyama.

Santosha – meaning contentment. How can you keep this feeling of contentment, even when things in your life may not be going so well? Can you still be open, relaxed and accept life as it is even when things are tough? Not condemning yourself for not being better or more successful than you perceive yourself to be.

Tapas – being disciplined even when things are difficult. For me, this is getting on my mat even when I am not in the mood, or I am feeling tired. The practice may not be the same and I will have to adapt, but it is about turning up for myself and seeing what happens.

Swadhyaya – study of self. This is about taking in knowledge through books, but also about reflecting on your habits and your ways of being. It requires honesty, awareness, and ahimsa (non-violence) to look at yourself without judgement or criticism. Not always easy to do.

Ishwar Pranidhan – surrendering to something bigger than you/God/Universe. This is about listening to your inner guidance and not being attached, and ego-driven. I equate this to the start of a yoga class where we set an intention, slow down, breathe with awareness and just start to listen to what is going on inside us. It can also represent the end of a class where we come into sav asana, letting our body rest, feeling sensations, emotions and allowing what is there to be there.

Asana

Asanas are yoga postures or as I like to call them, shapes you create with your body. This is the physical part of yoga and the third part of the framework and probably what most people are familiar with. There are hundreds of asanas, all designed to bring your body into harmony again in lots of ways. Some of the postures you may recognise in their English translation are mountain pose (Tadasana) tree pose, (Vriksasana) warrior 2 (Virabhadrasana 2) forward fold (Uttanasana) and of course, downward dog (Adho Mukha Svanasana)

When you physically align your body and move in and out of each posture safely, in flow with your breath, you can bring yourself back into balance again. Every asana moves our spine in a different direction and a healthy spine where all our nerves and energy channels (called nadis) flow to, is a super important part of a healthy body. "You are only as old as your spine," one of my many teachers said to me a long time ago and has stayed with me since. Asana practice not only releases space in the body, but it also prepares your body to be comfortable to sit for periods of time in meditation. It does this by releasing stuck energy and allowing the life force or prana to move freely through the body. When this happens, you feel better, move better, think better, breathe better, and lead better, allowing you to make better choices in everything you do.

Pranayama

Pranayama is breathe control. For me, this is the true magic of yoga and took my understanding to a completely new level. It is the reason I became a teacher. I like to think of your breath as being the link that connects your mind to your body. Your breath has a direct effect on your nervous system and can change the way you feel very quickly. During the asana part of yoga, synchronising the postures with the breath is what I teach during a class which makes the practice sometimes feel like a moving meditation. Pranayama is a practice all of its own and can be done before or after asanas. When you realise the power in your breath, you realise the power in yourself and all that you are capable of. It was a game-changer for me.

Pratyahara

Withdrawl of the senses. Our senses, especially in the world these days are stimulated and taking in information all the time. We get constantly distracted by the outside world and our mind races with thoughts continually over and over. Pratyahara is a practice of drawing all that energy back into ourselves. I always imagine it coming back into my spine and lighting it up as it lands there. This can be so challenging as distractions are always going to be there but recognising that and understanding how you respond to them is where the learning is.

Dharana

Concentration on one point. Here you focus your mind on one point or one thing. On average, you have over seventy thousand thoughts passing through your mind on any given day, so your mood should be relaxed and easy if you are to focus. The more frustrated and angrier you get, the less likely you are to succeed. I love to use my breath as my point of focus and eventually, my mind gives up trying to distract me and I can be fully in the moment with every breath. Sometimes I will use a mantra, which is a sentence or chant you repeat out loud or silently in your head.

It might be five seconds the first time you successfully focus on one point and that is ok. The next time it maybe ten seconds, but it gets better every time. Therefore, it is called a practice.

Dhyana
Meditation. Unlike Dharana where you focus on a single point, when you practice Dhyana, you merge with or become the object of your focus, bringing the mind into a beautiful state of calmness. All distractions from outside and inside are no more. This is the final preparation for the last limb of yoga.

Samadhi
Union of the soul and spirit. This is where you are in a state of complete oneness with everything and here you achieve a wonderful state of conncctcd bliss. My first experience with reaching this bliss happened at my teacher training course and one I will never forget.

Types Of Yoga And What To Expect At A Class
I am not sure how many types or styles of yoga there are, but there is something for every single body. You may recognise some of these ones: Hatha Yoga, Ashtanga Yoga, Restorative Yoga, Yin Yoga, Anusara Yoga, Kundalini Yoga.

My training was excellent and covered aspects from a lot of these styles. My classes are mostly from the Hatha style or classical yoga, focusing on alignment and safety, moving from one shape to the other and using the breath to get you there. Some postures are held for a few breaths and some for longer. I include pranayama, mantra, sometimes music and always a lovely long savasana, (relaxation) at the end of class. This is my favourite bit but sometimes the hardest bit! Finding comfort in being still and quiet can be so challenging when you have a million and one things going on in your head.

If it is your first class you may or may not need your own mat, some teachers will supply them for the class. Wear something comfortable that you can be relaxed in and move in. Give the teacher a call or drop him/her message with any questions you have. Look at the mat as your space. Nothing outside of this space should take your focus, except maybe the teacher! We are all human so I know this can be difficult, but comparing your practice to others can slowly allow self-doubt and feelings of not being good enough to creep in. In life, everyone is on their own journey, some ahead of you, some behind you. Yoga is no different and everyone starts at the beginning. Some days I feel I know little and still have so much more to learn about my practice and that keeps me forever the student.

Go with an open mind. Be kind to yourself. Be happy not being able to touch your toes or get the breath count right. It does not matter. One of my many teachers over the years said that the hardest thing about yoga is simply turning up. So just turn up for yourself, listen to YOUR body and see what happens.

Summary

As human beings, we are all going to face things in our lives that affect us and maybe even change us. Yoga gets you out of your headspace and brings you into your heart space. In my experience, people need to *feel* more, (heart space), not analyse or put into a box, (headspace), but feel all the feelings, good and bad. Only then can we let them move through our body as they are meant to. Children are our greatest teachers here and one of the reasons I went on to teach children's yoga. They have no filter when it comes to how they are feeling and express themselves, even though they may not know the words. Yoga teaches every age to feel, understand and name their feelings and to make better choices. The road to wellbeing and healing old wounds is about allowing these hard feelings to be present and let them move through us, so they are not ignored or buried. It will almost certainly be messy (there will be tears) and the reasons why lots of us do not do it. The other side of it though is great freedom and clarity, understanding of our incredible bodies, of ourselves and how we are connected to everything.

Yoga is one of the many things that can help you on your road to wellbeing and finding the practice that works for you is the key. Everyone is unique, so finding *your yoga* and what works for you is worth taking the time to explore. Please do not give up on it. Try several different classes, several different teachers, until you find the one that is right. A six-week course is not a quick fix, but consistency, practice, patience, and a lot of compassion will go a long way. On my own road to wellbeing, I have tried many styles of yoga and many other therapies; all have had their place, and all have healed and helped me so much. I was initiated as a Reiki therapist by Sharon Fitzmaurice and find Reiki truly healing and is a beautiful addition to the end of my yoga class.

Yoga makes you more aware of everything, who you really are, what is happening in your inner world, your posture, your food choices, people you surround yourself with, your thoughts and your emotions. I am a better person when I practice regularly, and my body will tell me when it is time to step back on the mat. Yoga is like my barometer for keeping me in check with my life. It could be yours too

Testimonials

I adore yoga! After years avoiding P.E and competitive sports, it's right up my street to move my body. I really feel all children should be introduced to it too. It does so much for me in terms of leaning into

the present moment on and off the mat. As a pharmacist, I dispense drugs to lower blood pressure, relieve pain, balance hormones, strengthen bones, reduce anxiety, manage depression and it always strikes me that yoga can help in every single one of these conditions without all the plethora of side effects. It's like a secret wonder drug we have had all along!- **Deirdre**

I am a mum of four young, busy lads and working full time. I found I was losing my temper, frustrated about everything and just not a nice person to be around. I did yoga when I was younger and enjoyed it, but then life got in the way and I stopped. My friend had worked with Suzanne as a coach and asked me to come to one of her classes to chill out! She was worried about me and told me she was afraid that something serious was going to happen. I loved the class straight away! It was hard at first to switch off, but her focus on breathing deeply in and out through the class really worked. The body scans are amazing, and my boys are getting used to me going" *all quiet "on them as they say. I look forward to the classes and just love the peace and quiet. -* **Catherine**

I signed up for yoga with Suzanne because my body was sore. I sit at a desk all day and get out for a run a few times a week. I find it hard to switch off, but I have learned ways to breathe that help. I miss it if I must work away and do not get to go to class. I had tried it before but just did not get it. Suzanne makes it easy to understand and although I still cannot do some of the moves, I am ok with it and do what I can. I always feel great after. - **Tony**

I started yoga during lockdown, following a recommendation from my next – door neighbour. I am forthy five and I do a lot of driving for my job. I am a psychologist. I mention that because you would think all psychologists are stress-free. Not so! The burden of the job can get to the best of us and it certainly gets to me at times. So, when I tried yoga with Suzanne, I discovered that my body had tension in places I did not know existed! Jeez, I thought, my body is crying out for this. Stretching and breathing is exactly what my body needs. I feel like my work is so much in the mind, but my body was ignored. Now for the first time, my body was being attended to, listened to. And it felt good. Now I practice short yoga sessions six times a week and I look forward to it. It is not a chore. It is a treat. Do not get me wrong it is not always easy, and I cannot touch my toes. But I can slowly feel my muscles stretching like elastic, tight elastic, but elastic. I am getting there. Thanks, so much Suzanne for giving me the gift of yoga.- **Suzie**

I had practised yoga over twenty years ago for a couple of years and took it up again in November 2019. It has been one of the best things I have ever done for myself. I started it again for physical reasons but realised within the first class the amazing mental health benefits. I practise regularly now, and it is an essential part of my well-being, especially as I am a working mom with children aged fourteen, eleven and nine. It was essential for me during the lockdown. I just know now that I will practise yoga for the rest of my life and it is going to be my refuge whenever the going gets tough; but also lovely and wonderful to do when life is good also, as yoga just makes life better. - **Aileen**

Recommended Resources

The Yoga Sutras of Patanjali if you want to know more:
The Body Keeps The Score, Dr Bessel Van der Kolk–super book to help understand effects of trauma on the mind and body
Change the way you look at things and the things you look at change
Dr Wayne Dyer, one of my favourite quotes ever!

My website www.suzannejoyclarke.com
Email info@suzannejoyclarke.com
Facebook https://www.facebook.com/coachyogabreath
Instagram @suzannejoyclarke

Finding My Voice
by Laura McDonald

My name is Laura McDonald. I live in Castlebar with my husband Joe, and four children aged twenty-one, ten, eight and five. I grew up in Wembley, North West London, and moved to Ireland in late 2006. I am a clinical hypnotherapist, BWRT® (Brain Working Recursive Therapy®) practitioner, Personal Trainer, and newly qualified Yoga Teacher. I have been in practice since 2004. I never really developed a strong sense of self. It is taken years of hard work to get an idea of who I really am and sometimes I am still not sure. There are many reasons for this; a cumulative sequence of traumatic life events from a young age which were subsequently compounded and reinforced time and time again.

I was born in London to my mother, who had left Ireland (Castlebar) after becoming pregnant. Mum was the daughter of a local doctor and the family were held in remarkably high regard. She and my father were not married, and society being the way it was back then, moving away was deemed the best thing to do. When I was two-years-old, my mum married the man I grew up calling 'Dad', and he legally adopted me. He already had two sons – my brothers – aged twelve and thirteen. A short while later, our sister was born. Dad was an extraordinarily successful builder, running his own business, and we grew up in a lovely big house that he kept extending and doing up. Mum and Dad had lots of friends and loved socialising and holding dinner parties. We visited Ireland regularly and spent time with Mum's family. Every year we spent the whole of August in Italy in Dad's hometown of Calabria, staying in a hotel on the beach, spending time with Dad's family, and holidayed in many other countries throughout the years. I played the piano, we went to Italian lessons, Brownies, had trampolining lessons, ballet lessons, went skiing with the school and more – we did not want for much at all.

However, we were encouraged to keep our ideas, thoughts, and opinions to ourselves, especially if they did not match the ideas, views, and opinions of those around us. We believed it was impolite, rude, or cheeky to speak up and we quickly learned not to. I cannot speak for my brothers or my sister, but for me, I felt a lot of confusion, wondering if there was something wrong with me for thinking differently, or feeling like a bad person if I had a differing opinion. I blended in and agreed and tried desperately to see things the way others did, no matter who they were. Polite and well-mannered, we did not argue or disagree, and generally were told to 'keep the peace'. It was not worth the alternative. I was discouraged from asking questions about my biological father and was not allowed to tell anyone, so I wondered lots in my own mind. Did he get married? Did I have other brothers and sisters? Did he think about me, did his parents think about me, did they even know I existed? … and so on.

I am a supervisor/mentor for other hypnotherapists and BWRT practitioners around the world. In 2016, I set up two training schools – one to teach hypnotherapy, and one to teach BWRT® to other health practitioners. My hypnotherapy school is currently the only one in Mayo, and my BWRT® training is the only training available throughout Ireland. I have trained in a few different modalities including reiki, EFT (tapping), facial reflexology, shamanic healing, personal training, yoga teaching, and more, but the ones I use at work are hypnotherapy and Brain

Working Recursive Therapy. Throughout writing this chapter, it has been challenging deciding what to share and what to keep private. I hope that what I have included gives some insight into what it is I do, some of the things I have had personal experience of, and how these therapies can help to make changes in your life, too.

I grew up finding it very difficult to speak up for myself in any situation. As I grew older and watched others expressing themselves and their views, I realised that everyone on the planet had their own thinking, and a right to express that. But by this time, it was so difficult to do. I was good at putting things down on paper and spent a lot of time writing. I know now that was a form of therapy, venting, and expressing my thoughts freely without judgement. Even now if I speak up, or ask for help, or tell someone something that does not suit, I still feel that guilt that I am inconveniencing someone else or coming across as rude. So, most of the time, I say nothing and get on with it.

I have too many memories of being called names. Stupid, strange, ugly, cheeky, rude, disrespectful, disappointing. The labels became a part of my identity – a self-fulfilling prophecy, and I really did believe them. My appearance was criticised, anything from my hairstyles, my eyes, my face, my skin tone, my posture — everything. I did not eat much when I was a child and I was teased for being very thin, too. I became convinced I looked odd, and that everyone was looking at me and thinking the same. If I were dressed up for a night out, I would often be told 'you should really put some lipstick on, you look unwell'. My confidence was always shot to pieces. Boyfriends did the same thing and chipped away at my confidence, to a point where I completely lost any part of myself that I had left. I was told what to wear, to cover myself up completely, every inch of flesh right down to my wrists. I was isolated from my friends. Once I tried to break up with a boyfriend and he laughed, looking me up and down saying 'who on earth do you think is going to go near you, the state of you! Do you really think anyone else would have you?' I have been pushed into furniture, thrown across rooms, dragged by my hair, spat on, and once pushed over in the street, cutting my head on the kerb. My serious lack of self-esteem had allowed this pattern to continue and while it made me sad, I did not even think anything of it. All I wanted was approval, so it just made me seek it more. It was not until I spoke to a therapist years later that I realised how messed up any of that was.

I enjoyed school, particularly all the sport we did, finding a great escape in it. Like most schools, we ran, played rounders, hockey, rugby, football, netball, basketball, trampolining, gym sessions. For the most part, I was a good student and threw myself into my studies. I had a fantastic group of friends who I am still friends with to this day. Living so close to Wembley Stadium meant we went to concerts all the time or sat outside and listened to whatever band or singer was playing at the time. We would spend weekends shopping on Oxford Street, weekday evenings cycling around the local park, and life was generally a lot of fun. When I got older, things started to change. I was diagnosed with depression at age seventeen, and no one really noticed or asked me what was wrong or why. My schoolwork started to suffer, and teachers started asking questions, but I just got told off and told to start getting my head back in the books. So, I did, got my GCSEs and finished school a couple of years later with five 'A' levels in English, Maths, Psychology, History of Art, and General Studies, and off I went to university, coming home at weekends for work.

One of the defining moments in my life was when I was pregnant with my oldest daughter. I was in the middle of studying my degree in English Linguistics and Literature and I had a part -time job three days a week. I was told that, I would never amount to anything. People told me I could not possibly do it all and that something would have to give – my degree or my job. Believing this (of course!), I went to my mentor at university and asked her advice. She asked me if I wanted to stop my degree, and I said no. She asked me if I wanted to stop working. I said no. She asked, 'why would you give up either, then?' Instead of being told what was best for me, what I should do, or what I could handle, I was asked what I wanted. I wanted to do it all – it was that simple.

I 'hid' my pregnancy from those who were disappointed in me, by wearing loose clothes and drawing as little attention to my bump as possible, so imagine my confusion when our baby girl was born and everyone rallied around, all excited and congratulating me. I did it all, continued with university and went back to work when our baby was four-months-old, and although challenging, it was fine. It taught me so much about effective time management, set me up for future challenges, and I started to believe my own strengths, abilities, and coping skills. I have pretty much continued to do things that way since. In fact, if anyone suggests that something isn't a good idea, or can't be done, it only encourages me to do it even more. These days, if I want to do something, I do it. I do not wait for 'the right time' or for a quieter schedule – I just do it. And I now have four children and a couple of businesses to juggle!

After completing my degree, I increased my hours at work while looking for suitable jobs. I signed up for a creative writing diploma course and a professional proofreading course. I was hoping to be a writer, speech therapist or teacher, and was thinking of completing a fourth year at university to do a PGCE. But looking through a newspaper one day, a familiar ad reappeared, one that my Mum had shown me years before, for a hypnotherapy course. She was more excited about it than I was, and I applied. It was a sixteen month course, one weekend a month, a twenty minute train journey away near Covent Garden. On the very first training weekend, I was so fascinated by the overall simplicity of the concepts of hypnosis, and I phoned my Mum on my lunch break, telling her all about it and that I knew this was what I would do; this was my vocation. That was in 2004, and I have not looked back since. As soon as I qualified, I started seeing pregnant smokers wishing to stop, in a clinic in Notting Hill, before setting up my first practice in a health centre in Willesden Green. After a year there, I moved to Ireland and settled in Mum's hometown of Castlebar. I started working in Kachina, a health centre in 2007 and am still there today. Since then, I have gone on to do hundreds of hours of CPD, and in 2016 opened my own Hypnotherapy training school, training others who wish to become hypnotherapists themselves.

What Is Hypnosis?

It is not what people often think. It is not one person having control over the mind of another. It is not 'woo-woo' stuff and will not make you do things you would not want to do. This is a question that is asked of every practitioner all over the world, and there are so many different views and definitions. My opinion is that hypnosis is a state of focus on a concept or idea, to the complete exclusion of anything else, and once learned, is a tool for life. It is a heightened responsiveness to suggestion and can produce a deeper contact with your emotional life, lift repressions and expose buried conflicts. It is a lifelong skill that once learnt, can bring about profound changes.

Some may call it an 'altered state', but that does not mean that you go into some strange way of being – rather, you become totally focussed on what it is you'd like to achieve, without any external interference from anything else: no doubts, no contradictions, no limiting beliefs. So, if I want to get up and talk on a stage in front of one hundred people, hypnosis will help me focus on doing just that. Visualising their faces full of interest, imagining myself full of confidence and in complete flow, imagining everyone there cannot wait to hear what I have to say, and filling the whole scene with motivation and excitement – instead of thinking 'I would love to have the confidence to do that, but I don't, I can't, I have nothing of interest to share, I am a terrible speaker, no one will be interested, what if I go red, what if I trip over, what if I forget my words….' What is happening in this second example is the same thing – but it is focusing on what I DON'T want. And the more we focus on what we DON'T want, the more likely we are to see that result because **the mind does not know the difference between what is real and what is imagined**. It takes it as a rehearsal – and if you practice well enough, you get what you picture. Therefore, so many sports people and athletes use visualisation – they visualise themselves scoring the goal. They visualise themselves running the fastest and reaching the finishing line first. They visualise themselves winning the game – they feel it all with every ounce of their being, they hear the sounds, and when it comes to the real thing, their strongly rehearsed visualisations start to play out. I teach every client how to use self-hypnosis as a tool for any area of life, not just for the issue they present to me with.

What Is Clinical Hypnotherapy?

Clinical Hypnotherapy is the therapeutic work that is done while one is in a state of hypnosis. We can communicate directly with the subconscious mind and make beneficial suggestions which will be accepted without argument. Providing we really want something,we can make it happen using this powerful technique. So, for someone who wishes to stop smoking, the hypnotherapy part is the suggestions that are made to stop them smoking. For someone suffering with low moods, hypnotherapy is the suggestions that they see the good in their life and the world around them, they sleep well, they have a sense of excitement about the days ahead. It is the focus on the beneficial sides of what someone wants, and the lack of argument from the logic part of the mind which says, 'you can't do that'.

How Has It Helped Me?

I could not possibly tell you all the ways Hypnotherapy has helped me. It has helped keep me calm in the most futile of circumstances and situations. As I said above, I grab opportunities as much as possible, because I know how they will increase my comfort zone, and there is nothing to really fear in going for things. Sometimes, I still cannot believe I opened a hypnotherapy training school, but the way I make decisions now is to ask myself 'would I regret *not* doing this?' If the answer is yes, I will give no more thought to it and I will take the plunge. Looking back now, I feel it was not actually a big deal at all, because my comfort zone has grown even more since.

Hypnotherapy has helped me realise why it was so difficult to start speaking up. When we are age 3 or 4, our sense of self/ identity is formed based upon the world around us. That is our reality/normality; what is real and normal for one person, will be quite different for another. Even though we grow up and realise we can think differently, the subconscious mind will not allow us to change that, because anything that is different is deemed 'unsafe', because it is unfamiliar. My low self-esteem led to an acceptance of being criticised by anyone who saw the opportunity. Because this is what the subconscious understood, it went on searching for, and only accepting, more of the same. While training, my mind went crazy with ideas, solutions, situations, people, and their problems, why people think and behave the way they do, why we repeat unhelpful patterns, why we accept things we say we do not want.

When the conscious mind and subconscious mind are in conflict, guess which one always wins? The subconscious mind. The good news is, we can change the subconscious programming. You can see a hypnotherapist, you can learn the art of self hypnosis, and you can plant anything you wish. If this were taught in schools, can you imagine the difference we would have in people's states of minds? Less bullying, less stress, more confidence, more understanding, and a world of far less conflicted people.

How Does It Work?

There are many ways to induce hypnosis. My preferred method is to guide the client into hypnosis using suggestion. I describe the concept of the conscious and subconscious mind. The conscious mind is the part we think with, talk with, reason with, and make decisions with – or so we believe. Our subconscious is all the stuff underneath–beneath the tip of the iceberg, and all our thoughts and behaviours are based upon what is stored in the subconscious. There is no logic or reason there – something either is, or is not. Its main function is to keep us 'safe', and by safe I mean to keep us in situations that are familiar, to make sure we always live according to what we know and understand. Anything that is new or unfamiliar is considered a danger, and is therefore to be avoided. We are not aware of what is going on, on a conscious level, which is why so many of us are constantly wondering why we cannot stop doing something, or why we find it so hard to do something new. With hypnosis, we can get to that subconscious part, make changes without the conscious mind interfering, and then wait and see the amazing results that follow.

As with any therapeutic intervention, hypnotherapy is not a magic wand. I have had clients come to see me in the past, thinking I can say a few things, and everything will miraculously change – but the work needs to be done by the client. I can only guide and advise. I remind them that I do not have control over them or their minds and that only they can do that. Commitment is required, as with any change, but the good thing about using hypnotherapy is that the changes that need to take place often become effortless, because we have done the work on the deeper levels of the mind rather than just surface level.

I start by taking a detailed case history from my clients to find out as much information as possible about them and their presenting issue. In some cases, I request consent from a GP and providing they agree, I can then put a plan in place as to how to best proceed. Provided you have a goal in sight, I can show you how you can reach that goal and what beliefs have been holding you back. Hypnotherapy can help you with countless issues such as smoking cessation; weight management; stress and anxiety; confidence, self-esteem and ego-strengthening; pregnancy, labour and childbirth and beyond; motivation; sports performance; exercise; clearing negative emotions and energy; some pain; healing the inner child; relationships, and so much more. I could write a lot about each issue, but for the purposes of this book I will summarise just a few:

Smoking Cessation

I love working with people who really want to stop smoking. Often, clients will call and say they have been smoking for so long, that it will not work, or that they smoke sixty a day, so it will be difficult, etc. This is not the case. However, for the hypnosis to be a success, I need my clients to really believe that, too — that it does not matter how long they have smoked for, or how many a day – it will work because they want it to. If they are stopping smoking because a spouse, friend, child or doctor has asked them to, it *could* affect the success rate, but if they are doing it because they want to, they are sick of it, they hate lighting up, it has a much higher chance of success.

There are three smoking cessation clients who still stand out in my mind after almost sixteen years in practice. My first smoking success was when I had just started my training, so I was probably three months into the course. He was a friend of mine and was so interested in hypnosis. I practiced with him and thought nothing more of it. A couple of days later, I sent a text to my friend, his girlfriend and asked her how he was getting on. I did not expect anything at all. To my complete surprise, she replied and said 'It's worked! He hasn't smoked since!' I was absolutely elated and even more excited about continuing this amazing training.

The next client that really stands out is a man who contacted me in my London clinic. He really wanted to stop but was concerned because his wife also smoked but had no wish to stop. Every evening, they would go out to the garden, smoke, and catch up on their days. He really did not want to lose that aspect of their day. I told him there was no need for that to go, that they could still go to the garden, talk about their day, and she would smoke, and he would not. He came for the appointment, left as a non-smoker, and to this day has never smoked again. He and his wife still chat in the garden, while she smokes, and he does not. His desire to be a non–smoker was so strong and has lasted ever since and it will for you too if that is what you *really* want.

The third client that completely amazed people around him was a man who smoked sixty a day and had had a triple heart bypass. His doctor had told him that he HAD to stop smoking or to expect the worst. Usually, if a client says their doctor requested it, I would sit with them and make sure they also really want to give up, and that it isn't just following 'doctor's orders' (because let's face it, we all know what is good for us and what isn't). This client had had such a fright with his health that he genuinely wanted to stop. He had said to me 'I'd love to be one of those people who sips water and picks at fruit all day' and laughed... I told him that is exactly what we would suggest.

A few months later, another smoking cessation client came to me and said "There's this guy at work, walks around picking at grapes and drinking gallons of water. He said he came to you, used to smoke hundreds of fags a day" and told me his name. Even though I never doubt the effectiveness of hypnosis, I was still quietly amazed but delighted. If you REALLY want to stop, it works.

Weight Management

There are many different reasons for weight gain; only some are about hunger or food. When I am contacted by people wanting to lose weight, I explain my approach, which is to look at the emotions, life events, relationship with themselves, and so on. In other words, we will be taking a close look into their psyche. The people who contact me are often those who have tried everything else, all the diets, all the slim shakes, all the clubs. Some have worked for a short time, but the weight has come back twice as much. This is because there is more going on here that needs to be addressed. As weight issues can be so complex, I wanted to offer more than just mindset, so qualified as a personal trainer with a qualification in nutrition for gym-based exercise. This is optional, of course, and clients can choose to exercise in a gym, or they might prefer a home-based exercise routine.

Clients are often eating to fill a void, and together we work to figure out what that void is. Many times, once we heal that pain, the weight sorts itself out as the client no longer finds themselves looking for comfort in snacking unnecessarily. I also share information on the best ways to eat (no distractions), what to eat, what not to eat, misleading information on what is considered 'healthy' and 'good for us', when to eat, when to stop eating, even down to how to chew food!

Inner Child Work

This is spectacularly healing work and something I have used for myself many times. Often our emotions can become stunted at the age we were when we experienced something upsetting. It does not have to have been something terrible – it can be anything that caused us overwhelm, such as losing a much loved toy. I have seen people start to cry when they talk about a minor childhood event and they're surprised that they can still trigger that sadness. Of course, often it *is* a traumatic event, but either way, we can 'visit' that inner child and tell her all the things she needed for comfort at that time. The domino effect of this can be astounding; it's almost as if we go back in time, fix something, and everything changes, no longer do we have that lost feeling and we feel more able to cope with whatever life has in store, feeling grounded and supported going forward.

Fertility, Pregnancy, Labour and Childbirth

I am a trained Fertile Body Method practitioner. This is a programme that can help some couples get into the best health for having a baby, by focusing on their lifestyle, nutrition, inner dialogue and much more. As with all physical issues, a letter from a GP will be obtained if they agree before any work is done.

I am trained in hypnosis for childbirth, and I have personal experience of pregnancy and childbirth both with and without hypnosis. Hypnosis for childbirth can help with fears, past traumatic birth experiences, and can help once the baby is born, reducing, or assisting with post-natal blues, tiredness, increasing sleep quality, even milk flow. As human beings, we are conditioned to believe childbirth is not a pleasant experience. We hear more negative birthing stories than positive ones, so naturally, there is a state of fear around childbirth. Hypnosis for childbirth trains the mind to remember that the body is designed to birth a baby, and it knows what to do, and it doesn't need any conscious interference so that when the time comes for the baby to be born, the conscious mind steps back and lets the body do its work. Hypnosis reduces the chances of tearing during childbirth, increases the speed of healing after childbirth, it can help with milk flow, it can help increase the quality of sleep in those first few months (or years) of getting up in the night, and can be invaluable in keeping the emotions in check when motherhood becomes overwhelming.

I had my first child before I trained as a hypnotherapist. I had an epidural. I requested it because I felt that is just what you do and it did not enter my head that I could try without it! Her labour was about eight hours long, which was good for a first baby. After she was born, I had two weeks of excruciating headaches to the point I could barely lift my head off the pillow. I am not sure for certain if that was down to the epidural or just one of those things.

With my second baby, about thirteen days before she was due, I had a few twinges. I had been practicing hypnosis for childbirth throughout the pregnancy, so I was not sure if the twinges were the real deal or not. I was on my way to work but called the hospital to explain what I was feeling. They told me to get my hospital bag and prepare to stay. I was calm enough to drive myself to the hospital and my husband met me there. Everything seemed so calm and controlled. When the pain became strong, I asked for an epidural, but they said I was too close to giving birth, and shortly after, she was born. I think I was in labour for a total of about three hours from the first feelings in the morning to the moment she was born. With hypnosis for childbirth, the mind is allowing the body to get on with what it is designed to do, without interference from the conscious mind, without fear so that labour can be going on with extraordinarily little pain or sensation. It is therefore important to let your doctors know you are having the therapy!

With my third baby, it was even faster. I had reached my due date with no signs of him arriving early as my first two girls had! I had gone up to bed and suddenly, about 11:30 pm, my waters broke. We went to the hospital and I was admitted to a ward and my husband was sent home. They said partners were not allowed to stay overnight and had thought I was not anywhere near giving birth. I kept calling the midwives to tell them I needed to be examined, but they did not think I was ready yet. Eventually, I convinced them I knew what was going on with my body, and when they checked me, the baby's head was already showing. They called my husband but by the time he arrived, I had already given birth to our baby boy, at 2:08 am. Again, it is so important to speak up and be heard… I was so calm and quiet they did not believe I could possibly be in labour, let alone fully dilated and ready to push!

With my fourth pregnancy, I was told quite early on that I had Group B strep. (streptococcus) This was obviously a concern as it can be extremely dangerous. The medical team advised me that it was a good thing to know so early on and that I would be given four hours of IV antibiotics during labour. I explained that my previous labours had been extremely fast and that I was worried I would not have time for the antibiotics, and they told me that if that were the case, the baby would have the antibiotics after birth instead. So, I had a few months to prepare mentally and had suggested to myself that it would be ideal to have longer labour than usual so that I could have the medicine the baby and I needed. I woke up one morning, eleven days early, just knowing the baby was on her way. We got to the hospital for 11 am, labour had started, the antibiotics were administered and almost four hours exactly later, my baby was born. It is important that I tell you I cannot say factually that the hypnosis slowed down the labour, but the doctors had all expressed surprise at my longer labour considering my previous babies had been so fast.

Illness, Grief, Bereavement

One morning, about twenty years ago, Dad walked into the kitchen. He looked different, his face had fallen on one side, and his posture seemed out of line. Mum and I asked him a few questions and his speech was slurred. He seemed to think everything was ok and was on his way out to work on a building site, so it was a challenge for us to get him to agree to be seen by a doctor. A stroke was confirmed, and he was never able to work or drive again. Everything changed overnight and so did he, usually such a strong, independent, able man now needing help from his family to do the simplest of things. As families do, we adapted and got through it, but a part of my Dad was gone, and this took a huge toll on his pride.

He has had two more strokes since, and his health has suffered tremendously, but all this meant that Dad has looked into some of the work that I do, and to my surprise, has asked me to help him on numerous occasions. Dad would not usually accept help from anyone, let alone treatments that are not considered 'conventional'. But he found great benefit in hypnosis, relaxation, and on occasion, even reiki! He even sought out acupuncture and found it highly beneficial. With my work, I have found this is quite common – that people will look for help only when something like illness has already struck. Dad lives on his own in London and while he needs a lot of help, he is still impressively independent considering what he has been through.

In 2007 we discovered our mum had breast cancer. I did a lot of hypnotherapy with her when I went home to visit, or when she came over to us, and she already knew how to do self-hypnosis, of course. She found it helped with her relaxation and de-stressing. She went through a gruelling treatment plan and thankfully got the all clear. However, early in 2011, the cancer returned. It was the year Joe and I were getting married. Mum was determined that the illness and treatment would not ruin her day and she was beside herself with excitement. Even though she was extremely ill on the day, sicker than she told us, she was beaming throughout. We were all hopeful that she would get better again, but she already knew that the cancer had spread.

In August of that year, I was told that my biological dad's health (who I had looked up when I was twenty-three and started growing a relationship with) had taken a turn for the worse and we were told he would pass away very soon. I spent as much time as I could at his bedside in the nursing home in Claremorris. One night, just after I had got home from visiting him, my aunt called to tell me he passed away shortly after I had said goodnight and left. Years' worth of sadness and tears poured out of me as I realised the enormity of everything that had happened, the feelings of grief and emptiness for a father I barcly knew. Maybe I was grieving for a life and a relationship we were never given an opportunity to have, maybe I was feeling the sadness he must have felt over the years.

The next morning, I woke up and realised I was bleeding quite heavily. I was six weeks pregnant with our third baby, so I went straight to the hospital and the doctors prepared us for the worst. I was taken for a scan, waiting for the news, until there it was, a little flicker of life right there on the screen. Our baby's heartbeat was healthy and strong. It was called a 'threatened miscarriage', often brought on by shock or stress, and I was told to take the rest of the pregnancy as easily as possible. I spent a lot of time working on my mind and body, telling myself all was well, my baby was strong, safe and healthy, as much as I possibly could.

I went to visit my family in London in October of 2011 and Mum did not seem herself. She was slurring her words, unable to eat properly, and seemed unsteady on her feet. I mentioned it to my sister, who reassured me that it was just the medication and that I was not used to seeing her that way. Mum had an appointment at the hospital, and we were dealt the worst news imaginable, that the cancer had spread into her brain and that we needed to prepare. We were under the impression we had a few months left with mum until the doctor looked us in the eyes and said it could be weeks. I will never forget having to tell Dad.

I went back to Ireland to sort out what I was going to do. I needed to organise the children, and Joe would need to take time off work if I were to move back to London to help care for Mum. I had no idea what to do or how I was going to do it. A day or two after, I returned home from being out to find Joe waiting for me on the doorstep. His face was white, and he did not speak. Instantly I knew it was Mum. 'Has she gone?' I asked.

'No, but we need to get to London tonight'. He had already booked a ferry and we needed to leave around 9 pm to get the 1 am Dublin ferry. Those hours were long and awful as neighbours and cousins came over to pay their condolences. She had not even passed away yet. The drive was the longest drive ever. I had that 'pull' that you need to be somewhere, but there is nothing you can do. We were on the ferry with our two girls, we slept in short shifts, and drove again on the other side to the hospital in Kensington & Chelsea. My sister had said on the phone that mum was not herself and did not recognise anyone around her. As we walked into the room, she turned to look at us. 'Who is this?' she said, looking at me. Her eyes moved to our oldest daughter and something shifted. Her face lit up with recognition in her eyes. 'My darling, come here,' she said, and opened her arms out in an embrace. Our daughter had totally brought her back and we spent six bittersweet days with mum in the hospital: Dad, me, my sister, our two brothers, our oldest daughter, and Mum's sister. Visitors came and went, we laughed, we cried, and she passed peacefully on 17th November, 1:30 am, the day after our second daughter's second birthday. I was now five months pregnant and holding on with every ounce of strength I had left. 'I must not break down. I must not break down,' was all I heard going through my mind, for fear of hurting the baby. I practiced self-hypnosis as often as I could possibly do it, telling my body it was doing an amazing job, it was healthy, it was strong, designed to carry a baby, a healthy happy baby, all the suggestions I could possibly think of.

Mental Pain

After our baby boy was born, everything seemed perfect on the surface, but underneath, I was drowning, without even realising it. Looking after three small children while grieving both my parents during pregnancy finally took its toll. The health nurse came over one day, and I presumed she was there to check the baby. She was there to check me because my husband had called her. She asked me a few questions and I remember answering, not really caring, nor wondering why. She booked me an appointment with my GP, who asked me some more questions, and I was diagnosed with depression again, prescribed anti-depressants and referred for six months of counselling.

Up until that point, I had not wanted to take anti-depressants, because as a therapist, I believed I should be able to sort my own head out, I did not need pills. This time, I was willing to do anything to get out of this darkness. It was not like the depression I had experienced before which had included extreme sadness. No, this time it was just nothing. I had no feelings, no sadness, no anger, just nothing. And that was scarier than anything. I always encourage my clients to follow their GP's advice – if you need medication, please take it! In my case, the anti-depressants helped lift me out of a hole, like a ladder over a fence. Once I could see the other side, I was equipped enough to carry on without them but that takes time.

Many of us know that there are often no visible signs of depression. I remember telling one of my close friends that I was going for counselling and was on medication, and she had been genuinely shocked. She said she had seen a photo I'd shared on social media days before, and commented on how happy I had looked. Throughout it all, I practiced self-hypnosis, even on days where I thought 'what's the f*cking point?' Discipline is key to taking care of ourselves, whether that be mentally, physically, or emotionally. Knowing the power of the mind is what kept me doing it. I knew that if I wallowed in my negative thinking that I would just feed it and make it bigger. Start with a few positive thoughts – ANYTHING – feed and water those ones instead and watch how things change. The mind is everything. If you would like to try a few simple hypnosis audios, follow my free collection on Insight Timer.

Physical Pain

About ten years ago, I began feeling pain in my feet. It was like walking on broken glass and was usually worse first thing in the morning. At first, I did not really take much notice, but then it started spreading to my ankles, knees, shoulders, elbows, and hands. It got so bad that I could not clench my fists, which meant I could not get dressed, shower, brush my teeth or do anything without chronic pain. It affected things that we take for granted, like cooking, driving, playing on the floor with the kids, holding them. I ended up in hospital on a few occasions, and an MRI showed five bulging discs, three in my spine and two in my neck. A blood test showed rheumatoid arthritis, and a DXA scan showed up osteopenia in the lower spine. I have done so much work on myself to help manage the psychological side of dealing with such horrendous pain, the worry about damage to my joints, the fact that it is considered a life-long illness that can flare up at any time. I take a strong medication which often leaves me feeling sick and tired a few days of the week, which is tough not just for me but for those around me.

My work has helped me to accept that I have this illness, manage it, and take care of my body in the best way I can. My recent yoga teacher training has been a huge help. I first started doing yoga over twenty years ago, not knowing what a profound effect it has on the mind as well as the body, and I am looking forward to incorporating it into my work, designing a range of different classes including those that help with pain, whether that be emotional, physical or both. The physical practice (asanas) is only a small part of yoga, with the main principle being that 'Yoga is the stilling of the fluctuations of the mind.' I have every belief that my physical ailments have an emotional root cause, and this is yet another area I am currently studying, but as with the depression I have found myself in, I will work alongside conventional medicine and keep up to date with my doctor's advice.

Emotional Pain

I had thought that moving to Ireland would be straightforward. We speak the same language after all – but it was not. I had come from a life of 5 am alarm clocks, 6 am underground commutes and 7 am starts in a city where no one really takes any notice of each other (we did not even know who lived across the road), to a town where everyone knows everyone. It was massively overwhelming and still can be, at times. I will always love and miss London, the anonymity, the busyness, the having things planned weeks in advance instead of last minute. But since I've learned to embrace things here, to slow down and adapt accordingly, things have started to shift. It is a totally different world in comparison, but one that really works for my family and me. There is less time rushing around and more time to be, which has allowed me to recognise the importance of really listening to the mind and body and resting accordingly. All too often, we are encouraged to wear the 'busy' badge of honour, and in my case, that busyness was sometimes me avoiding what was really going on. All go, ignore, ignore, ignore. I used to work constantly, or meet with friends, have hardly any sleep, all because I could not face what was going on in the depths of my own mind. But eventually, it all came crashing down and things needed to be dealt with in the end. I realised I was stealing from myself – and have learned in my yoga studies that one of the Eight Limbs of Yoga teaches us to be aware of that:

Asteya–a–*not*, steya – *stealing.* Do not steal from others, whether it be possessions, time, or energy. Do not steal from the self; be gentle in practice, do not push yourselves into postures you are not able to do. Likewise, do not allow others to steal from you whether that be possessions, time, or energy.

This was an eye-opener for me. As human beings, we naturally want others to be ok, and as a therapist, it is my job to help people find a place of peace. However, it often overflowed in my personal life (and already had throughout childhood), with people offloading all their problems on to me and asking for advice. I never saw it as an issue until I learned this word (asteya) and realised how much I was giving and allowing to be taken from me. I would be messaging friends while my children were trying to talk to me (stealing from *them*), for example, or sharing advice when it was me that needed rescuing.

As a wife, a mother of four, and a therapist, I owe it to my family and my clients to be in the best possible place to be able to take the best care of them. More importantly, I owe it to myself. We all know the saying 'you can't pour from an empty cup' and there are no truer words; this goes for each one of us! We need to learn to tune in, listen, and behave accordingly. Being still is not lazy, nor is it unproductive. It is quite the opposite, and wonderful revelations and ideas come when the mind can be still. It is a treatment that I offer people, called 'emotional clearing', where clients come in and switch off, while I create suggestions that clear their minds, their bodies, their souls of all negative emotional energies. We spend so much time cleaning our houses, our bodies, our clothes, our possessions, but we spend nowhere near enough time doing the same for our minds. Can you imagine how much more productive we would be if we made it a priority to do that? Our confidence, clarity, capabilities, and state of mind would go through the roof. All by taking a few moments each day, just being. We would free up so much more time because the work we would be doing would be ten times as brilliant without all the negative energy and chit chat going on in the background.

I want to give people hope, that no matter what they are dealing with, no matter how long for, they can come to a place of peace, and to give them the tools to manage to maintain that peace. I do my best to convey this message to my children, too. It is hard to find a balance, but I hope I am getting there. I encourage them to work hard, but also that it is important to sit back with a book and a blanket when the mind needs time out. I allow space for them to become bored, as it is a perfect opportunity for them to come up with something to entertain themselves and so important too. I teach them to be patient; they cannot always have what they want, when they want it, because otherwise, how will they cope in the big wide world when they realise nothing comes to us easily? I do my best to sit with them, ask them how they are feeling, if there's anything bothering them, remind them that they can tell us anything, let them know that no one can treat them in a way that makes them feel uncomfortable, and so on. At the same time, if one of them is acting up or throwing a tantrum, I try to look at it asking myself 'What's going on for them right now?' recognising that this is often coming from a place of pain, anger, fear or frustration. Of course, sometimes it is simply just bad behaviour and it will not be tolerated…! But my message is, if I add fuel to the fire by losing my temper as well, it is only going to exacerbate the situation. I've been in situations where the children are fighting by 8 am and the whole day has been ruined because they're angry, I am angry, my work suffers, and we go around in circles until bedtime, and other days where I have dealt with the situation calmly and it's changed the whole course of the day.

Brain Working Recursive Therapy – What Is It?

Now, for something exciting. As a requirement of my role as a therapist, I do regular CPD, which I absolutely love. I have done countless courses, but nothing has stood out to me as much as BWRT® (Brain Working Recursive Therapy). I studied it in 2014 and it is a technique like no other. It is not hypnosis, energy work, NLP, or anything like anything at all. It's a model of psychology and psychotherapy created by UK professional therapist, Terence Watts. It allows a 'core of privacy' so that you do not have to divulge anything you would rather not talk about.

BWRT® is based on the latest discoveries about the way the brain works and how it affects our moods, behaviour, and emotions. It works with the reptilian complex of the brain, and we can effectively 'rewire' our neural pathways and change our responses to practically anything at all. This has been monumental in my practice and I became busier than ever. As with any business, there is a lot of work behind the scenes – and a lot of mine is working with new students, helping them pass their exams, and mentoring licensed practitioners online, anywhere in the world. I also offer the only practitioner training available in Ireland.

I can still remember my very first BWRT® client and the look on her face when she realised her presenting issue had disappeared. I am not sure who was more excited – her or me. From then on, I practiced it on friends, family, clients, word started to spread, and the enquiries came flooding in. It is not unusual for me to have a waiting list of five to six weeks because people are so excited about it. One of the things that clients love is that there is no need to go delving into the past, nor is there a need to tell me anything they would rather I did not know, or they would rather not talk about. We also do not need to know where the issue came from. We can just get to work on the uncomfortable feelings straight away.

There are different levels of BWRT®, which work with different ranges of issues. Level 1 works predominantly with all manner of anxiety, stress, confidence, fears, phobias and allows the core of privacy. Levels 2 and 3 require more in-depth knowledge of the client and their presenting issue. My most memorable Level 1 client was a young man (shared with permission) who was so anxious, he could not leave his bedroom. After our first online meeting, he was able to eat dinner downstairs with his family. After four sessions he was going for drives, going to family gatherings, organising his twenty-first birthday party, and the last time we were in contact he had moved out of the family home and set up his own business.

I have used BWRT® to help people with trauma, abuse, jealousy, anger, confidence issues, weight issues, chocolate addiction, alcohol issues, and a lot of sports people. I regularly work with professional tennis players, runners, and high jumpers who all describe the same performance anxiety; everything is great while training, but when it comes to actual tournaments, races or competitions, the nerves take over. The results have been phenomenal, allowing them to reach their full potential and beyond. I have worked with professional singers and DJs with mental blocks when it comes to writing material or performing on stage. I have helped victims of bullying to build back their confidence, whether it is bullying from school days or even in the workplace. I've also helped fear of heights, claustrophobia, fear of public transport, fear of lifts, fear of water and swimming, chronic fear of needles, fear of flying, fear of spiders and other insects, fear of dogs, fear of school, discomfort around certain people, fear of social situations, as well as exam stress. In fact, some students dislike certain subjects so much so that their mind does not allow them to focus on revision; but BWRT® can change that! BWRT® is having particularly amazing results in the townships in South Africa and is the favoured therapeutic intervention for the highest qualified psychologists and psychotherapists dealing with the most complex and traumatic events in people's lives.

At the time of writing, I am enrolled on a BWRT® course called Neurophysical Enhancement Therapy, which I am extremely excited to introduce into my work. As the name suggests, the programme uses psychology to focus as many neurones in the brain and body as possible to enhance physical performance and endurance. It will enhance body fitness, strength, health and longevity and I cannot wait to introduce this to my sports clients, those wishing to increase health and fitness, or those who may want to add a daily walk into their regime.

I love hypnotherapy and BWRT® in equal measures, and both offer a quite different experience for the client. Some people want their issue dealt with super-fast, with no need to talk about it or even tell me what it is. Others want the relaxation aspect that I include in my hypnotherapy sessions; the music, the candles, the dim lights, and a feeling of lightness they can carry around long after. Both work extremely effectively, or I would not use them at all.

If you are dealing with something in your life that you are ready to let go of, or you feel is holding you back, you can change it. Sometimes we become so used to things that we believe it is just the way we are and that is that. We hold on to limiting beliefs and restrict ourselves from taking chances. This could not be further from the truth. If you have a clear idea of how you would like to be, or how you would like to feel, then these techniques can really help. If you are not yet sure how you would like to feel or what goals you have in place, wait until you know just what it is you want until you think about trying these techniques. When you are clear, you will be committed and motivated to getting stuck in and doing the work and it will be a far greater success!

Overall, my approach is to encourage people to embrace the holistic outlook, treating the whole person, the mind, the body, and the soul. We should look after our minds and bodies as a daily routine, the way we shower and brush our teeth without thought, instead of waiting until something goes wrong. No matter what clients come to see me for, I always throw in a good dose of confidence–building. All parts of us are interconnected and if the mind is healthy and strong, the body is healthy and strong; when one suffers, so does the other. My work with exercise, yoga, and my experience with mental, emotional, and physical illnesses are all testament to that. Exercise is as much therapy for the mind as it is for the body and it is no secret that people feel great after exercising, whether that be a full body workout or a walk around the block.

Thank you so much for reading my chapter. There is so much more I could say, and I hope to share more with you sometime in the future. I love that I can schedule my work around my husband and family. I see clients when my children are at school, I run courses on the weekends, and I do my mentoring, administration, and voice recordings late into the night when everyone else is asleep. I get the best of both worlds running my businesses to suit the family and getting to do the school drop-offs and pick-ups and cook dinner in the evenings. If there is anything you are wondering about or something you think hypnotherapy or BWRT® could help, please do get in touch.

Every therapist has their own style of working, so what works for me and my clients is not necessarily what will work for another practitioner and theirs. There is no one way to do things. When I teach my students, I give them all the necessary tools and let them decide which ones they will use, and which ones do not suit their practice. They bring their own personalities and life experience into their work so that there is a therapist for everyone. My hypnotherapy courses are open to anybody who has a strong desire to learn more, whether that be for personal use, professional use, or both. My BWRT® courses worldwide are available to those who are already health practitioners, but there is a course available for the complete newcomer, listed on the official website below.

You can find out more about my work and other techniques I have experience with on my websites here:

- Eden Wellness www.edenwellness.ie
- E.I.C.H. Ireland (Hypnotherapy Diploma Practitioner Training) www.eichireland.ie
- BWRT Ireland (Therapy and Courses) www.bwrtireland.ie

All 3 businesses can be found on Facebook, Twitter, LinkedIn, Instagram and others. https://linktr.ee/LauraMcDonald
Listen to my free hypnosis audios/Yoga Nidras on the Insight Timer http://insig.ht/edenwellness
Contact me at laura@edenwellness.ie

I Never Lost Hope
by Mariona Duignan

My name is Mariona. I am living in Galway, but I am originally from Girona, a city to the north of Barcelona. Some people cannot understand why I have been living in Ireland for so long. You can imagine it is not thanks to the weather... From time to time I balance the 'pros' and 'cons' of staying in Ireland and if the 'pros' win, I don't make plans to leave. I do not know if I will always live here. What I miss the most are my sister, my family, and my closest friends that many times were more supportive than my family. I also miss the heat of the sun, the taste of the food, the smell of Mediterranean Sea, the Catalan and Spanish live music, and many other little things that Ireland never will be able to give me. Girona is a beautiful city, only thirty minutes away from the beach and the mountains.

I am married to Adrian, an amazing man from Roscommon and we have a beautiful daughter. I feel incredibly lucky I met him; he brings so much joy into my life. I believe we make a very good team and complement each other very well. He is great craic and I like to laugh a lot. What I admire the most in him is his ability to simplify problems and to look at the bright side of everything. Together we try our best to have fun and enjoy the little things in life.

I did not have an easy childhood. I come from a dysfunctional family. My mum has been struggling with mental health issues all her life. I was the first daughter, and I always tried my best to please my parents. I could sense my mother's sadness and I always tried to bring happiness to her. Now I understand that this role was not healthy for me, but I did not know it before. I could see my dad was very worried about her. He used to talk to the doctors and psychiatrists about her; according to them, she was never going to recover from her disease. The diagnosis was chronic depression and the prognosis was not optimistic at all. Doctors always said that my mother was never going to be healthy. I used to get terribly angry about 'this life sentence'. How could they know about my mum's future? Why could they not give her any hope to recover? If none of them believed in her recovery, how was she going to find healing? Why nobody tried to understand the emotions hidden in her depression to help her to build a hopeful future?

I could not understand it and looked for answers. I used to read my parents books from a Catalan psychiatrist called Doctor Corbella. I was only ten years old, and I loved reading books that were bringing some light to people's problems. Since I was very young, I have been attracted to how the mind works. My husband says that I am addicted to self-help books. And in some way it is true, I always look for solutions when I feel down or anxious. I always loved reading people's stories of recovery because they give us hope and they teach us that after a bad time it will get better. There is no way around it. We all go through difficult moments and we come out of them. Nobody has a great life all the time; we go through ups and downs. This is part of our journey as human beings.

Some people like to show that their life is always perfect, but this is not possible. And the efforts to keep up the pretence of being happy is wasted energy. It would be much better to use this energy to feel the emotions you have to feel, whether it is sadness, anger, panic, fear, anxiety, grief, worry, etc. and just trusting that they will pass. I know they are unpleasant feelings, but they are necessary for our healing. If we try not to feel any emotion and we mask them with alcohol, tobacco, keeping busy all the time, watching Netflix, taking legal or illegal drugs, we are never going to heal them, and they will come back sooner or later. I believe that we are here, on Earth, to grow and to experience what it is to be human, and we only have one life to do that. Since I was young, I could hear my mum crying and shouting a lot. I did not understand the reason, so I always looked for support in my dad. He used to explain to me what was going on with my mother.

My mother is an extremely intelligent, overly sensitive, and emotional woman. My dad is a very rational man, quite grounded and good at looking for practical solutions. He taught me how to enjoy the little things in life and I am very grateful for that. I learnt from my mum to never give up when I do not feel well. She is the person I know that has done the most to feel better. She has looked for healing in many different types of therapies. She eats a very healthy and balanced diet. She does everything she is told to get better, but she is still struggling a lot. And many times, I think that this is not fair…she deserves a better life. Myself, my sister, and my uncle still hope that she will get better…

My mum told me that I had an 'easy birth'. It was on a Saturday and people were celebrating carnival. She felt a few strange sensations, went to the hospital at noon and they told her to go home and come back at 3 pm and around 6 pm I was born. She said that my birth was exactly how she read in the books. She told me that she felt a lot of joy. My sister's birth was even easier; it just happened in three hours from the beginning until the end (that is what my mum says).

My first memory is from when I was two-and-a-half years old. I was on a plane between my parents going to Menorca. I remember the excitement of 'flying' and that a hostess gave me sweets.

My second oldest memory is a little bit more traumatic. It was the day before my fourth birthday. I was (and I am still) a very stubborn child. I wanted to make orange juice. My mum was busy in the kitchen and she did not want to help me to make it, so I jumped onto a chair to start making it, but I slipped and a pot full of boiling water burnt my left arm. I do not remember the pain, but I do remember the fear. My biggest fear was to go in an ambulance. My dad was not at home, so my mum had to ring an ambulance. I was incredibly lucky that my dad arrived home before the ambulance and he brought me to the hospital. It was a serious burn, a third-degree burn. The doctor put me in plaster to immobilize my arm for a few weeks. My mum had to take time off to look after me. I remember we had a nice time at home, playing lots with my mother.

During my childhood, I was a very good student and athlete. When I was five-years-old, I was in a sports club where I was practicing four types of sports: basketball, tennis, athletics, and gymnastics. After two years of doing these sports, we had to pick one. My favourite was gymnastics. I was very flexible, and I loved being connected to my body. The gymnastics' teacher wanted me in her team, and she gave me the highest mark (ten out of ten). I really wanted to join it, but my parents decided that it would be healthier for me to do basketball because it is a team sport. They thought that if I joined the gymnastics team, I would be 'too cool for school'. They considered that the pressure of training and the professional competitions would be too much for me (and possibly for them as well). I got very angry when my parents forbade me to join the gymnastics team. I felt they did not listen to me. I could not understand their reasons. Now, thinking back I realise that I made so many good friends in the basketball team, I am still in contact with many of them. Many times, I realise that when things do not go the way we wish, it is for our highest good. There is a lesson behind every frustration, a blessing in disguise.

When I was ten years old, I was bullied in school. I suppose I was the typical nerd. I always knew the right answers and a couple of people did not like me in the class — they were probably jealous. I was the class rep, and I used to shine. I had many friends and I was enjoying life fully. My mother was a teacher in the same school. My mother talked to my teacher, and she said that it was not clear that these two guys were bullying me and said I was provoking them. I remember I used to feel threatened and I used to cry every evening at home. My parents decided to changed me to a different school. The new school was a private school, closer to our home. I used to walk with my sister to the school. I was ten years old and Marta was four years old. I loved her to bits, but she was a nightmare. She was trying to make the journey from home to the school and vice versa quite complicated. I imagine she was only a child looking for my attention. She used to lie in the middle of the road, pull her skirt up at any moment, she would ask me the same stupid questions every day, embarrass me in front of my new friends, etc. The new school was nice, they made me the class rep in the first year.

I consider myself quite a friendly person, easy-going, kind, funny, sensitive, positive, smiley and with lots of energy. I have all these qualities on a good day. When I have a bad day, I am the opposite: a little bit rude, dry, profoundly serious, anxious, and sometimes I find hard to stop thinking negatively. I suppose you better catch me on a good day!

The new school was a nice fresh start for me. I joined the basketball team of the girls that were one year older than me and I was still a very good player. I made friends for life — some of them came to my wedding last year!

When I was around five or six years old, my parents enrolled me in a music school. I have lots of good memories. My grandad used to collect me in the school and bring me to "El Tamborí". The best part of the music school was that there was no pressure, no exams, no marks, and no homework. We used to play and learn and make friends. After a couple of years, we had to choose one instrument. I wanted to play the piano. My parents tried to change my mind; a piano was quite expensive to buy. They tried to persuade me to play the guitar, the flute, or any other instrument a little bit cheaper but my stubborn mind wanted a piano. And after fighting for a year, I got the piano. I still remember my first piano teacher, a particularly good pianist. Playing the piano was an escape for me. I absolutely loved it. Music has always been a life -saver for me. I played the piano until I was seventeen years old. Then I stopped because I felt guilty that my parents were paying for a teacher and I was not studying at all at home.

The piano always brings sweet/sour memories... I am incredibly lucky that I have my piano in Galway, my uncle posted it as a wedding present. To be honest, I had no time to play much since the piano is in Galway, but I am hoping that I will be able to play when my daughter is older.

My granny Montserrat (my mum's mum) carried a lot of grief. Her dad died when she was five years old when there was the Civil War in Spain (1936–1939). My granny Montserrat was the youngest of five and she was separated from her mother and siblings because of the war. She was well looked after by her uncles, but she felt abandoned by her mum while grieving the death of her dad. Two uncles were killed because they were priests. She never recovered from that. She constantly talked about how hard it was to live in these conditions. She was in strong physical health but mentally and emotionally she was in pieces. Not able to live in the present moment, always remembering the shadows of the past. I remember my granny shouting quite often for no reason. My grandad used to tell me: '*Just think she is like a storm, she will shout and then will pass...*'. And then she was caring, she loved playing table games like domino, cards, and monopoly, she was good cook and used to sing while cleaning the house.

My granny Montserrat was one of my study cases in my last year of homeopathy. She was diagnosed with dementia at eighty-six years old. She was under homeopathic treatment for five months with me and then I referred her to a more experienced homeopath in Barcelona who treated her until she died last February. During the homeopathic treatment she had overall improvement of her aggressive and violent behaviours. Irritability, anger, feelings of being dominated, suspicious, fear of robbery and desire for company improved over the first four months on a single homeopathic remedy. She stopped perceiving the reality as dangerous and threatening. However, the loss of memory and general disorientation were still apparent. Then I prescribed a deeper remedy that brought some positivity in her life as she was able to feel thankful and did not feel dominated by others.

Every time I went to Girona, Adrian and I went to visit her in the nursing home. I thought it was very funny one time that one of the carers told me: '*I love your granny; she is such a peaceful woman!*' In my opinion, homeopathy helped her to heal the trauma of living in a country in war and the disease helped her to forget the worst memories. Just thinking in a romantic way, her funeral was on the 14th of February 2020, when I believe she joined again her beloved husband (my grandad Santiago) in another place. They never celebrated Valentine's day because in Catalunya we have another tradition for lovers on the 23rd of April when men give roses to the women they love, and women gives books to the men they love.

When I was seventeen years old, I was diagnosed with depression. My parents were very worried about me because I had no energy for anything. My dad brought me to one of the most popular psychiatrists in Catalunya — Doctor Corbella. He prescribed some tablets and he recommended that I go to a psychologist. I did psychoanalytic therapy for seven years. It helped a lot to find my own truth and to identify what problems were mine and what problems were coming from the people around me that I was absorbing. It was tough, because the whole perception of what was going on my mind kept changing session by session. At the same time, it was very positive for me because I found my roots and my essence. I had a strong desire to leave my family and my country for long time. I felt strongly that I had to leave to heal myself, to save myself. I left behind many friends that were as important as my family. It was sad, incredibly sad for them and for me, but the desire to have a better life was stronger. I keep in touch with most of them, I still love them so much and love to connect when we can.

During the summer of 2006, after finishing a Chemical Engineering Degree, I worked in a bank and I saved a bit of money to come to Ireland. My mother gave me some extra money to do an English course. I desperately needed it because my English was terrible. In September 2006 I moved to Ireland. I came on my own, but I knew that two weeks after, my friend Ruth would come to Galway for a few months. I was living in the Barnacles hostel in Shop Street and studying English in the Atlantic School. Soon after, I found a job in an Internet Café (*Chaternet*). It was a challenge to run a shop with phones and computers on my own. It was great 'craic'; we were a lovely team of young people spread in different shops in Galway city. I made lots of friends and I enjoyed talking to people every day.

After one year I found a better paid job in a medical factory and I saved money to travel around the world with two of my colleagues from work. We bought an open ticket to South East of Asia, Australia, and Hong Kong. I remember this trip with a sweet/sour taste because just a couple of days after booking my flights, I met an Irish guy (my current husband). To be honest I was quite annoyed about 'having to travel' when I just was starting to have a nice relationship with a man. My heart wanted to stay a bit longer in Galway to see how our relationship was going to develop. He had travelled a lot before, and he wanted me to go. I could not understand why he was pushing me so much to travel. I used to feel so small, I thought that probably he did not like me as much as I liked him. But life is like that, I was with him for five months and I decided to jump into a new adventure again. Although I found it very difficult, we kept in touch every week and when I went back to Galway, he was waiting for me in the bus station.

I studied a course of massage, aromatherapy, and reflexology in the GMIT. It was a two year course, but I only did one year. I really liked it, but I felt it was not for me because I was exhausted after giving three massages a day, so I thought that it would be quite difficult to make a living out of it. Then I found a job as an administrator. The job was ok, but I didn't feel very welcome or appreciated.

Due to the stress that this job was causing me, I used to get Shiatsu massages. One day the therapist told me: *'For the type of problems you are telling me, I would highly recommend you to go to a homeopath that practices in Salthill, Sara Howlin'.* The first time she told me this, I did not follow her advice. One year later, she repeated, *'I think that a homeopath could really help you because it has helped me in similar problems.'*

I made an appointment with Sara and I believe that much deeper healing took place. I felt 'listened to'. During the first consultation she took a detailed care of my anxiety and insomnia symptoms as well as my family history and struggles. I felt safe, I felt in good hands. She did not say much, she let me talk, she did not give me any advice. I remember she told me '*I'm going to light a candle for you to find a better job*'. She only gave me one remedy to take under the tongue, and she recommended me to book another consultation after six weeks. I remember her gentleness. I felt she was holding my hand to walk with me for a while, a proper hand.

Around one year after being under homeopathic treatment, the situation at work was still complicated. I really wanted to leave this job. I had a couple of interviews in pharmaceutical and engineering companies, but no luck. No doors were opening for me. During one of the sessions I explained to Sara that I had a strong inner feeling that I wanted to change my professional career. I felt that I wanted to study something related to health, maybe homeopathy. Sara told me about the Irish School of Homeopathy, the only accredited school in Ireland to study homeopathy. I attended a six-week course that they organised in Galway. We had very inspiring teachers, and very grounded information. I connected very quick to it. All I wanted was to learn more and more so it did not take me long to decide that I wanted to study homeopathy professionally.

In September 2012, I started the four-year professional course in homeopathy in Dublin, and my life started to change profoundly. I stepped into a journey of studying and learning that has never ended.

There has always been great support from the teachers, tutors, supervisors, and directors from the school. I was blessed to be in an amazing class with beautiful people from many different countries. We had a wonderful time, we learnt in an atmosphere of joy. We were known as the 'giddy class' because we laughed as much as we studied. In this class I met Tonia, a wise woman that has helped me in many levels. We formed a study group. We complement each other very well. We were the only ones from the West of Ireland, so we travelled together to Dublin every month. I am so grateful she is still an important person in my life. Now we run homeopathy workshops together.

Homeopathy is a natural system of medicine that treats the entire person. It works by stimulating the body's ability to heal itself; homeopathy supports your immune system. Homeopathic remedies are made from plants, animals, and minerals in homeopathic pharmacies. Rather than treating one part of the body or one single symptom in isolation, homeopathy takes a holistic approach and considers the total symptom picture of the person — physical, mental, emotional, and spiritual.

Physical health can be described as freedom of pain, health of cells and organs, fitness level and flexibility. Emotional health involves freedom of expression, self-acceptance, ability to give and receive love, self-awareness, acceptance of thoughts ability to be in the now. Mental health is the ability to deal with difficulties and problems, focus, clarity of thoughts, ability to make decisions and to be spontaneous. Spiritual health can be considered the ability to enjoy life, appreciation, gratitude, awareness, the ability to meditate and feeling a purpose in life. The ideal is to have a balance between the four types of health. Some people may only have many physical ailments but feel incredibly happy themselves. Other may suffer from emotional problems without any physical complaints. All these variables are taken into the equation when the homeopath chooses the potency of the homeopathic remedy.

The process of analysis of a case and the selection of a remedy is quite complex. After a first consultation, sometimes my clients need to wait a few days to receive their remedy. This is because I take my job very seriously and I do not prescribe any remedy unless I am sure. I work with other professional homeopaths and we support each other in difficult cases (always protecting the confidentiality of our clients).

Remedies can be taken in different potencies. The potency refers to the dilution and the 'strength' of the remedy. It is indicated by the number and the letter following the name of the remedy, i.e. 6c, 30c, 200c, etc. For home prescribing, usually potencies of up to 30c are most appropriate.

Homeopathy was discovered by a medical doctor from Germany named Samuel Hahnemann (1755–1843). In an attempt to understand why cinchona bark (china) was successful in the treatment of malaria, he repeatedly ingested the substance and found that he developed the symptoms of the disease. This refers to the first principle of homeopathy — 'like cures like'; which means that a disease can be cured by a substance that can produce similar symptoms in a healthy person. This principle can be tracked back to Hippocrates (known as the father of medicine) two thousand years ago and further developed by Hahnemann.

Hahnemann discovered that when a substance is diluted in steps with forceful shaking (succussion), the therapeutic effect is not only retained but is enhanced, without any toxicity. This process of dilution and succussion is referred to as 'potentization', which makes it an energy medicine.

There are different types of prescribing. This is a very complicated field which keeps evolving with the years. To make it simple, there are three main types of prescribing: first aid, acute and constitutional. First aid applies when the remedy fits the situation i.e. shock, accidents, fright, burns, sports injuries, etc. Acute prescribing is when the remedy fits their symptoms, modalities and/or cause. Constitutional prescribing is when the remedy fits the person and their disease. Only professional homeopaths can prescribe constitutionally.

It's quite easy to learn to use homeopathy at home for minor ailments. The main variables to take into consideration are: concomitants, location, aetiology, modalities and sensations (known as CLAMS). For example, if we have a cough, the concomitants would be any other symptoms that you are also having with the cough, such as shivering, fever, sore throat, etc. The aetiology is the cause of the problem; for example you may have developed a cough after being outside and getting very cold. The modalities are what makes you feel better or worse. When having a cough, some people may feel better drinking hot drinks, while others may prefer cold liquids. The sensations are what you feel in your throat, i.e. tickling, dry, etc. So as you can see, the remedy is selected case by case.

Some clients don't understand why different homeopaths would prescribe different remedies. It's very easy to understand. When we are looking at a persons' case, it's like looking at a tree. I may be looking at a tree from the left side, while another homeopath may be doing it from the front. So we just see different perspectives of the same tree. It's very important not to expect quick results. If you have been suffering from a chronic illness for many years, your healing is going to take time. I always tell my clients to give at least three sessions to evaluate if the treatment is working (although many times improvements are noticeable a couple of weeks after taking the remedy).

Personally, I think that the essential element in an individual's healing is the connection with the therapist. It's very important that you feel safe and able to open up with your homeopath. If you are hiding information, the homeopathic treatment is not going to work and I would recommend that you change to another homeopath or another therapy that doesn't involve talking.

In January 2016, I went to Mumbai with a group of homeopaths from Ireland to learn in-depth a method developed by Dr Rajan Sankaran: The Sensations Method. It was an incredible experience. My homeopath, Anne Irwin has a lot of experience in this method, she studied with Dr Sankaran many years ago in Goa. Homeopathy is like everything: it keeps evolving and thank god there have been many gifted homeopaths (apart from Hahnemann). I have a very deep connection with the Sensations method because it has worked very well for me. It has been a crucial part of my healing journey and it is an essential tool in my practice.

When I was one month pregnant, I joined The Dream Team, a group of extraordinarily successful homeopaths that were looking for help in their project. A few years ago, they created a course online to teach mums how to treat minor ailments at home, such as colds, flus, coughs, digestive issues, etc. At the same time, they were offering a free support group online seven days a week. I was part of this support group. It was a privilege to witness how mums were empowered to heal their own families. On some level, I think it was perfect for me because it gave me so much experience prescribing acute ailments and the possibility to connect with a group of professional women that tried their best to support each other. The group of mums was named The Home Prescribers Rockstars, a very cool and encouraging name.

The Dream Team has two leaders: Rita Kara Robinson and Antoinette McWeeney. They are a 'cracking team', I see them as real soulmates because they complement each other very well, and there is a lot of love, respect, and companionship between them. They are pure magic together, able to come up with innovative ideas to keep evolving and growing.

When I was two months pregnant, I joined a 'business course' online created by Antoinette and Rita (The Love Fest). I am grateful for all that I learnt during these six months. We were a group of twenty three homeopaths, all women. We grew together; we are still growing, some together, some apart. This course helped me to recover so much confidence in myself. I reconnect to my own power. Between the pregnancy hormones and this group of women, I felt my energy coming back bit by bit. They taught me that when women raise each other, we are powerful. They taught me how to navigate the cyclic nature of being a woman. There were lots of different meditations and activities. I can say that I came out stronger and feeling supported. In ways, all the 'work' I did for the year was giving noticeable results.

I felt great most of my pregnancy. I felt strong, grounded, worthy, lucky, loved, and productive.

Very soon after finishing this course, my daughter was born and a whole new dimension opened: motherhood. I stopped focusing on my healing and started focusing on the wellbeing of my daughter. Of course, always taking care of myself in order to be the best mum I could be for her. I do not always get it right, but I do try my best, so does Adrian.

Homeopathy can support a wide variety of diseases. There are two more cases that I would like to share with the permission of my clients. I have changed their names to protect the privacy and no personal details are given.

Mary came to me a few years ago. She was sixty-seven years of age. Her main complaints were stiffness of hips (especially the right hip), general stiffness first thing in the morning, aching bones, cracking joints (knees, shoulders, feet, and fingers), watery eyes (worse in the morning), tendency to break bones and anxious dreams. She was under homeopathic treatment for five months. She has an improvement of ninety percent of her stiffness over the first three months on a single remedy. Cracking joints, watery eyes and aching bones improved seventy-five percent during this period. Stiffness in her feet in the morning got completely better. She felt calmer and her anxious dreams disappeared.

Kai, a seventeen-months-old child was diagnosed with prolonged bronchiolitis. He started crèche when he was one and he developed the following symptoms: a wheezing chest, rattling respiration, congested nose, couldn't breathe properly, cough with green phlegm worse in the morning (sounded like whooping cough), vomiting, recurrent chest infections, recurrent ear and throat infections. His doctor prescribed nine rounds of antibiotics and two rounds of steroids, but there was no long-term improvement. After two days on the homeopathic remedy, his mother reported a noticeable improvement of the symptoms. Six weeks later, his mother said that wheeze was gone, rattling respiration was gone and that the biggest change was the release of chestiness. Kai was feeling good.

Homeopathy has survived over two hundred years despite the deliberate bad publicity that certain people impose on it. If homeopathy was 'crap', it would not be available in so many countries and used by so many millions of people. We are not stupid, and testimonials speak for themselves.

After writing this chapter, I have realised the power of vulnerability and how strong and healthy I am. Thanks to homeopathy and all the people that have supported me along my healing journey.

Facebook @marionaduignanhomeopathy
Instagram @marionaduignanhomeopathy
http://www.marionaduignanhomeopathy.ie/
marionaduignanhomeopathy@gmail.com
PH: 085 2428663

Finding My Feet
by Therese O'Reilly

My name is Therese O'Reilly. I am a lot of things, wife, mother, daughter, sister, friend, holistic therapist, reflexologist and some would say a 'mad yoke'. But who am I? Before I even start writing, I am gripped with fear of sounding like an 'eejit!' The little red fella on one shoulder is screaming 'Why would anyone give a damn about your story!' and the little angelic one on the other shoulder is whispering 'You're amazing, you've come so far, just write!' So today, I am going to try to overcome that fear and share at least the bits of my life that got me to here and how reflexology has been a constant for me for the last twenty-two years. They say everyone has a book in them so hopefully, I will be able to squeeze out a chapter.

Born and raised in the West of Ireland, the fifth child of seven I had a happy-go-lucky uneventful existence, free from any real hardship and free from any fear of judgement. I simply did not notice if I was liked or disliked. I was just me. I was a happy child. I just went with the flow. We all worked hard on the little farm. I started work at the age of thirteen in the local hospital, at weekends and holidays. Although some of the nuns in the hospital could be quite vicious, I used to feel sorry for them. I enjoyed the elderly patients and would sing to myself as I worked. I remember a nun got terribly angry at me one day. I was humming or singing doing my work when she screamed "Why are you always so happy? I'll fix you". She had me scrub the bathroom floor with a toothbrush and soapy water. She did not bother me. I just did it. I enjoyed nature and did not mind all the hand-me-downs. I trained as a chef after secondary school and immediately thereafter headed to the big smoke at age nineteen. My attitude remained the same, happy, and hardworking, although I did sometimes feel lonely there. In my early twenties, I headed to New York for six months. The six months flew by and turned into a year, then two, three and so on. I ended living in New York for twenty years. For me, New York was an adventurous city, a massive melting pot steeped in culture and other manifestations of intellectual and musical achievement. There was always something to do, somewhere to go. My cooking skills served me well and I was never unemployed.

My first encounter with despair came when a lad I was going with for a couple of years went off with my friend. Although I knew this relationship was not right and would never last, the ending was not on my terms. It was abrupt and painful. For the first time, I had experienced betrayal, self-doubt, and heartbreak. I lost the boy, but I also lost a friend. Rod Stewart was so right about the first cut being the deepest. But it did not kill me, and I recovered. I mention this because in hindsight, the ending of those two relationships was the beginning of a marvellous journey of self-help, discovery, and resilience. To escape from the pain, I went back to college, working multiple jobs to pay for it, cooking in the mornings, waitressing and bartending at night. I became a paralegal. I threw myself into the arts, going to plays, concerts and galleries and explored the city. I eagerly devoured every self-help book I could get my hands on. I came to believe that the Universe had my back and every insignificant seemingly unimportant thing happened for a reason. I thank God for that two-timing boy and the fake friend.

So, I had my qualification but I didn't know how to break into the legal profession in New York City, when I had no connections. Well, as it happens, in one of the restaurants I worked in, we had a very grumpy regular customer that nobody wanted to serve, including me at the beginning. I ended up serving this old man every day for months. We eventually warmed up to each other and in between his complaints about the food, the weather, etc. we talked. I challenged his views on the world and politics. We had great conversations and I found him interesting. He would ask me why I was waitressing and what did I want to do in my life. What I did not know for ages was this man owned his own law firm and ultimately offered me a job. This was the man who gave me my start in the legal profession, which I worked in for about fifteen years. I still remember the feeling the first day I took the bus to his office in the South Bronx, over by Yankee Stadium. I was most definitely the new girl on the block and stuck out like a sore thumb. Terrified and excited at the same time.

Life was exciting. I lived in the Bronx and had my own apartment. I think everyone should live alone for a while. It gives breathing room and atmosphere to grow. After some experience, I got a job in Manhattan. I slowly clawed myself up the ladder to a decent salary. I worked in my last law firm for ten years. I travelled to London, Chicago, Vegas, and Miami while working with this company. I worked hard and enjoyed it. I met a great new fella Seamus, my now husband of nearly twenty-five years. We moved into Manhattan — two blocks from the Rockefeller Centre for a few years. We had a blast. It was exciting to live in Manhattan in the heart of it all — St Patrick's Cathedral a couple of blocks in one direction, Central Park a few blocks in another. I walked to work, wore designer clothes, lived high on the hog without a care in the world. In our early thirty's we started a family and moved to an outer borough.

Our first pregnancy was a miscarriage. It was a difficult experience for us both and the sadness hit us hard. We went on to have three healthy children and at age thirty-five I had a boy and two girls. There were eleven and a half months between the last two, Irish twins! I thoroughly enjoyed three healthy pregnancies. I loved been pregnant. It was not that every minute was pure bliss, but there were moments of pure transcendence, unlike any other time in my life. I was healthy and happy and felt truly alive and full of vitality. It was during my pregnancies that I accidentally discovered reflexology, although I did not know it was reflexology at the time. My feet were constantly sore, so I would sit on the couch at night and rub them. I noticed the change of tissue texture when I put pressure on my feet, a bit like popping bubble wrap.

I heard it said the three biggest events in your life are getting married, having a baby and buying a house. Well the day I came home from the hospital with our youngest, we moved into our new house. Three c-sections in five years, a toddler, two babies, a new house and a full-time demanding job — it was not long before the shit hit the fan. On the outside, I smiled and acknowledged my great life, but on the inside, I was totally overwhelmed. I felt like I was being dragged into a sinkhole. I constantly thought my head was going to burst with the pressure. All the lessons I learned from all the self-help books swam around my head confirming that I just could not cope. I cried a lot. My husband did not understand what the heck was wrong with me and neither did I. I had never heard of post-natal depression. I loved my little family so much, but my anxiety was through the roof, I could not sleep, I could not think, I would get agitated at the drop of a hat. I did not enjoy being around people, and I worried that I was a bad mother, an inadequate wife. It was totally crap and I suffered a lot. I hid my feelings from my husband and friends for a long time and felt totally alone.

One day, at the paediatrician's office I just let it all out. I had accidentally cut my daughter's finger when cutting her tiny fingernails. In my head, I had committed a crime and was completely distraught. I was inconsolable. The paediatrician was an older experienced lady and quickly recognised that this was not just about the fingernail. She was so wise, kind and understanding. She comforted me and assisted me in getting the help that I needed. One of the therapies I turned to at that time was reflexology. It was so relaxing. Reflexology eased my anxiety. I slept better, the agitation ceased. I had weekly treatments for some time. As I slowly returned to myself, I spaced out the treatments and went on a maintenance plan. It was at that time that I knew that I would practice reflexology myself one day.

Thankfully, life got back on an even keel and time marched on. While still living in New York and the children were quite young I injured my back, herniating a couple of discs. It was very painful and debilitating. My consultant advised not to have surgery as I was a young woman and he said my back would never be the same again if had the surgery. So, I opted for physio, exercise, and reflexology. I was amazed at how my pain levels dropped after a session of reflexology. I could stand up straight and walk with ease. Severe pain can take over your life. I cannot stress enough how important it is to get a handle on it. It can change a person. When it comes to pain, sometimes the cure can be worse than the disease as tablets can totally disrupt the digestive system. I tried the painkillers for a while but had to dump them rapidly, as my system just stopped working. This also happened many years later with another injury when I suffered from a frozen shoulder, another excruciating painful diagnosis. I could not take the pills, so I went the holistic route with regular reflexology treatments. By the time I had the shoulder injury, I was practicing reflexology myself and could do daily hand reflexology treatments. It really saved me by lowering the pain, especially after surgery and helped me get back on my feet.

In 2008, after twenty years in New York for me, twenty-five for Seamus, we moved back to Ireland. We returned to our Celtic roots from our adventures and experiences in New York City to reconnect to our homeland and beloved families. Looking back, it was such an epic undertaking. The amount of work involved was massive. Leaving a life that we worked years to create and starting all over — it just blows my mind when I think back. Setting up in Ireland was no easy task. Trying to get information and figure things out was an arduous task. As luck would have it, the whole economy crashed shortly after we arrived home. We moved into a small cottage, no jobs, no prospects. Disaster! We decided to stick it out as we felt this was the right choice for us and we slowly got going.

Despite my fears, this time was transformational for me. Letting go was not easy, especially when I was used to thinking a certain way about my life and how to live it. I had to release old ideas and embrace change so I could live my best life. There is a tendency to expect the worst when the first signs of difficulty arise, but by taking on the challenge and going through the temporary discomfort, it all comes right in the end. It was during this time that I decided to re-educate and among other things I enrolled in a reflexology course. I dived into my studies with clear intentions, practising and reading any book I could find. I had to complete sixty case studies before qualifying. I loved it and devoured all the information. So, back on my feet, I was on the road again, happy out with my little family, moving forward. Helping people made me happy.

Returning to my hometown after twenty years, I was a person of interest, at least for a while! I was new. Some welcomed me back with open arms, some with cautious curiosity. I was outspoken, did not conform to dogmatic small-town society. So many people wore masks all the time — smiles on their faces and sadness and suspicion in their eyes. I probably did the same myself. I would hang out and chat, socialize with people, but felt empty after. When you have been away for a long time; it is hard to break back in. I was the friend that came home for two weeks every year, the friend to stay with for a shopping trip to New York. People had formed their tight friend groups, and although they would talk, they were not really letting you in. There was no craic. I longed for authenticity. I was drawn to different women's groups and meditation groups. I have learned more about friendships by returning home from New York than ever before. One of the most important lessons I learned is to never put anyone on a pedestal because they will fall off! And, unfortunately, not all friendships survive the demise of the pedestal. No-one is perfect and in true friendship, you should not have to be. A wise girl shared one of her mom's sayings with me, 'True friends are like diamonds, precious and rare, false friends are like leaves, found everywhere'. I suppose as I get older, I realise that it is less important to have lots of friends and more important to have real ones.

The worst period of my life was four years after I moved home from New York, and my father died suddenly. People commented about his great age and long life, but the pain of grief was profound. It was the darkest time of my life. I experienced the many stages of grief, the shock and denial, the pain, the guilt, the anger, the fog. I knew grief was the natural response to the loss, but I did not expect the huge physical, mental, and even spiritual effects that I went through. And I could not shake it. Depression crept in slowly. I withdrew. Nobody noticed.

The fair-weathered friends disappeared rapidly. When I cried, they could not cope. As often happens after death, my original family endured the first of many family breakdowns, a long and arduous story for another time.

Totally disillusioned, suffering from heavy grief without the support of friends and family, my mental health began to deteriorate. Depression is quiet and is easily disguised for a while. The cheerier you are, the less people see. I felt stressed all the time and my anxiety grew. The persistent, unshakable dark feelings haunted me. Everything felt like pressure. I had no pleasure or enjoyment even in the things the I loved. I struggled on my own for a long time. I had to write things down because I could not think. I had trouble focusing or thinking clearly. The fog was deep. I tried to pull myself out of it by running, but the tiredness was massive. I used to run the county roads with a couple of girls. If the roads were quiet, I would run between them with my eyes closed. I would listen to their banter and laughing. Thank God for those girls. They just accepted me the way I was. Maybe they knew I was not myself, but they never said. They just flanked me and protected me on the road. The fatigue was overwhelming at times. I had no problem sleeping, in fact, I could have slept all the time, but I had a young family, I had to keep going. I unintentionally lost weight. Everyone said I looked great.

Feeling very alone and helpless, my thoughts became morbid. I lost my perspective and often contemplated a permanent solution. Thinking this way offered me some temporary relief. I talked to my doctor. Suicidal Ideation she called it and assured me I was not at risk, that it was a coping mechanism. I believed her. I did not want my brain thinking this way, so I tried to help myself. I completed a suicide awareness course and suicide assist course. During the course, we had to role play. When I finished, I got a clap and a couple of people had tears in their eyes. My heart was pounding because what they did not know is that for me, it felt so real. I was trying to keep myself alive.

To make an awfully long story short, I suffered like this for about three years. Thankfully, after one remarkably close call,

I finally resolved to get help. I could not continue the way I was. The mental sink hole was wide open, and the continual downward swirl was like gravity sucking me in. My foundation was not solid anymore and I was truly at risk. I knew that I had not the strength to swim against that tide for much longer. The swirl was getting faster and the pull greater. I sought help again. Desperate for a solution to my problems, I went for counselling and turned to holistic therapy once again. I trained in reiki and became a reiki master. I returned to my beloved reflexology with a vengeance, helping people like myself who were struggling to cope? I went on retreats searching for my old self. I also trained in Indian Head Massage and I set up my own meditation group. I learned that you could clean the outside of the glass, but if you do not clean the inside you will not achieve the clarity you seek.

I learned that nobody was going to come and rescue me, but when I decided to rescue myself, there was an abundance of amazing people there to assist me. I learned that keeping quiet is the silent killer that can lead to stress which left unchecked can lead to anxiety and not dealt with can lead to full-blown depression. Depression can be a lonely and dangerous place.

I remember the day I shared my experiences with a group of twenty women at one of Sharon's retreats in Bog hill. My heart was pounding, and my mouth was dry as it was my turn to share. I had been on a few retreats before and shared bits of my life but never this. I thought I was going to choke with the lump in my throat, as I spat it out and my mouth went like sandpaper. When I finished, you could hear a pin drop in the room. I had finally said it after years. Nobody knew only my husband, my niece, and my sister-in-law. It was like a weight was lifted off my shoulders, my chest, my heart. The room was completely silent.

Sharon thanked me for sharing with a twinkle in her eye as someone handed me a tissue. In the next breath, she asked anyone in the room who had a similar experience if they wished to, to raise their hands. Almost a third of the people in the room raised their hands. I could not believe it. I thought I was alone, and no-one would understand.

My point for sharing these very personal experiences in my life with whoever is reading this is You Are Not Alone! A problem shared, no matter how big or small, can diminish and sharing can help to lessen its power over your whole body, mind, and soul. I lost myself for a while and that is ok. I got back on my feet, more than once. Nobody is perfect. We are all a work in progress. I still get lost from time to time. My driving force, my passion and motivation has always been my family; my husband, my son, and my daughters. When I would go on the retreats and when Sharon would ask what is your passion, my answer was always the same, my children. They are all big now and do not need me in the same way anymore, a transition that is not the easiest for me. It is time for me to step back and let them be, give them room to flourish and trust that I have done my job. I will always be their role model and their biggest cheer-leader.

I decided to step into my own power, find my purpose, stand on my own two feet again. I learned that everything is energy and it is my choice to only accept positive energy. My power comes from my connection to my own consciousness and the universe and my self-worth. I learned from my suffering, my emotional ups and downs. My breakthrough was to genuinely love myself again, the way I did when I was a child. The only way I can inspire any of you to love yourselves and take care of yourselves is to love myself. So again, I return to what fulfils me, helping others, through reflexology and other therapies.

What Is Reflexology And Where Does It Come From?

In a nutshell, reflexology is a theory and therapy that uses the feet to treat the whole body. Reflexology is ancient art and science that practices the principle that there are reflex areas in the feet and hands that correspond to all organs, glands, and body parts. The unique method of using the thumb and fingers to apply pressure to these reflex areas in the feet, hands, ears and more recently the face. This sends a message through the body to the corresponding organ.

The body is highly intelligent and knows how to heal itself, but it needs to be in a balanced state to be able to do so. Reflexology helps in that process to bring the body to a state of homeostasis or balance, so then it can heal.

There is evidence through ancient tomb drawings in Egypt, India, and China that reflexology dates back as far as 2330 B.C. These drawings show a person holding another person's foot and applying pressure to the soles. This supports a form of hand and foot therapy in ancient times, in the pyramid of Ankmahor, also known as the 'physician's tomb' in Egypt. It was also practised by American Indians and African tribes. Reflexology transformed over several centuries before coming West and becoming what it is today. In the early 1900s a very interesting America called Dr. William Fitzgerald, who was an Ear, Nose and Throat surgeon developed the zone theory. This was the theory between reflex zones in the feet and hands corresponding to different parts of the body. His research was carried on and further developed by lady called Eunice Ingham.

Eunice Ingham was a physiotherapist from South Dakota. It was Eunice's research earned her the fond title as 'Mother of Reflexology'. Reflexology became her passion and she had the courage to pursue it. She spent much time studying the feet and analysing tender spots in relation to the anatomy. She discovered that the reflexes on the feet are a mirror image of all the organs and charted the first map still used in reflexology today. She developed the unique thumb and finger movements that reflexologists use today. Eunice wrote the first book on reflexology entitled *'Stories the Feet Can Tell Thru Reflexology'*. In her book, she talks about the crystal in the nerve endings in the feet and her explanation of uric acid build-up, as well as many other aspects of reflexology. Eunice travelled the world giving seminars about reflexology. She was a pioneer of reflexology. She dedicated her life to reflexology and helping people. After she retired in the 1970s, her nephew Dwight Byers formed the International Institute of Reflexology and continues her work to this day.

Who can reflexology help and what are the benefits of reflexology? Eunice Ingham believed that reflexology could help mankind and I agree with her. Simply put, reflexology can help everyone. Although it is not used to diagnose or cure disease, millions of people around the world use reflexology to complement other treatments. One of the biggest benefits of a treatment is relaxation. It improves blood circulation, relieves tension and induces relaxation and rest, uplifting the mood. Reflexology is a great stress management tool. There is an endless A–Z list of conditions that can be assisted by reflexology from asthma, constipation, headache, hormonal imbalance, pain, sciatica, and the list goes on.

For example, if a person comes to me feeling sluggish, low energy and complaining about not being able to lose weight, I will treat the whole foot but may pay a little more attention to the thyroid gland which will, in turn, help with the functioning of the metabolism, balancing it and thus aiding weight problems. It will also help to bring metabolism back into equilibrium.

Working on different parts of the body through the feet is beneficial to everyone. Working on the adrenal reflexes helps imbalances in the hormonal system. They are also important for treating any stress-related disorders and inflammatory conditions. Working on the kidneys reflexes benefits the whole excretion process, making it more efficient. The kidneys are also one of the reflexes I would work on to help regulate blood pressure, as the kidneys purify all the blood in the body.

For anyone with lowered immunity, I would concentrate on the liver which detoxifies, also the lymphatic system and the spleen which help fight infection. For back pain, I would work on the spinal reflex. My clients range in age from two years old to eighty years. I treat young people stressed out from studying for exams, young couples trying to conceive, babies with teething, men with sciatica. Reflexology is for everyone and can be used to help with any condition. It is a complementary therapy that can be used alongside traditional medicine.

Although I do energy work, reflexology if a physical therapy with proven physical results. A treatment with me consists of a short consultation and you lie on the therapy couch. I prefer to do a silent treatment so that you can just totally relax and reap all the benefits of the treatment. Clients are grateful for not having to chat or make small talk. I am a hundred percent focused on the person I am treating, so I can uncover what the feet are showing.

In conclusion, I loved and lost a few times, I suffered, I recovered. I am resilient, I am the only superhero in my life. The only gift I have for the world is to let my light shine. My passion and purpose are to help as many people as I can to take care of themselves. I do this through reflexology and energy work. I appreciate every day that I am alive, and I appreciate all the amazing people who have helped me along the way. I have learned from all my experiences, the good and the bad. Fear is just an illusion. If I can teach my children, one thing it is resilience. Life's hard. You have to bounce back and land on your feet. I no longer accept or take on other people's negativity. Other people's crap is just that, their crap. Love me or do not. That is up to you. Decide to be happy. One last thing I have learned is that you never know when you going to meet a real friend. It is priceless when you do. I encourage you to be kind to each other and let your light shine. The world needs what you have to offer.

085 7722684
Tuam Reflexology & Master Reiki
therese_oreilly@yahoo.com
www.reflexology.ie

Emotional Freedom
by Nuala McCann

My name is Nuala McCann. I found this weird and wonderful technique called EFT back in 2010. I'd like to share with you how I came to learn this technique and how it has helped me and others. Back in 2003 I was working in a medical device company in Galway City. I really enjoyed my work. I loved learning new things. The pay was great, and I got to meet lots of new people, which is something I really like to do. After about four years and a series of unfortunate events at work, I had had enough. I remember standing in the cleanroom with my mop cap and gown on and thinking "Is this it? Is this all there is?" I had outgrown my job.

I had started my own awakening journey when I attended my first ever workshop called The Healing Angels of the Energy Field back in 2005. It was my first introduction into the Angelic Realms. I bought my first deck of Angel Cards and I was fascinated by the messages I would receive. It was around this time that I met Sharon Fitzmaurice. I would attend some of the Angel Meditation mornings at her home. It was great to meet others who I could talk to about Angels. It was also around this time that I found the work of Abraham Hicks. This was my first introduction to the Law of Attraction. I also came across Esther Hicks in the original version of The Secret movie in 2006. I've been listening to them ever since.

I continued at my job in Galway, and I worked through different shifts, departments and roles for three years following that workshop. I had a workstation where it was just myself and on some days, one other person. At random times throughout the day, I would have people pull up in the chair next to me and start chatting. They often had something that was bothering them, and they just felt like sharing it with me. This was a regular occurrence and I really enjoyed it. It helped to pass the time at work too!

One day someone (I can't recall who it was) said to me after one of our chats, "I always feel so much better after talking to you. Have you ever thought of doing this for a living?" I really want to thank this person for asking me that question. It led me on a path that I never knew existed and I know that question was heaven sent. The answer was no. I had not thought about it at all. I never thought that I could make a living out of doing something that came so naturally to me.

Don't you have to do things that you do not particularly like in order to earn money? Making money is hard right? (False beliefs right there!) I pondered this person's question and I really do not remember how it happened but, in 2008 I enrolled in a foundation course called Foundation in the Humanistic Approach to Counselling/Psychotherapy. I was always fascinated by people and how they thought, what they did and what they would say. I thought "Well if I'm good at listening and helping people feel better, then I'll get certified and become a therapist". Perfect. I had it sussed. Go me!

Unfortunately, I hated it. I loved the learning and the self-reflection, etc. but I hated the practice sessions with clients. It did not make sense to me. In Talk Therapy, we have a client talk about what they are struggling with. We help them find a new perspective, give them ways to cope and manage their situation or help them come to terms with a traumatic event they had been through. Ultimately have them be OK with where they are and take steps to help themselves out of the situation. It can take many sessions before the client gets any significant relief from the emotional aspect of the issue.

The part I hated was that when the client was talking about their issue, they would inevitably start to FEEL the emotions around it. Now, I have been for therapy before. So, I know it is not possible unless you have really trained yourself not to feel anything, to tell your story WITHOUT feeling any emotion. So, I would start talking about what was going on for me. I would feel the emotions I had about it, I would try to come to an understanding about it, but I would be left feeling very raw emotionally at the end of the session. What was I going to do now? Where do I put these emotions? My session was over. I had to go home to my kids. Help with homework, make dinner, and connect with them. But inside I was an emotional wreck. All I wanted to do was to go to sleep to switch off my feelings. But that was not an option for me. I had three kids to take care of. So, I would stuff my emotions back down and get on with life until the following week. I decided that if that is how I felt then others must be experiencing this too. I thought "There has to be a better way than this". A way that is less traumatic.

I know that Talk Therapy works. It works for a lot of people and I think it has its place in the healing world. But personally, I think it can be done in a way where the client does not have to experience the feelings to such a degree that they fear talking about their issue. That is why most people do not seek therapy. They are trying to avoid how they feel because the original event was so traumatic. The thought of going back there is scary. So, I gave up on the idea of becoming a psychotherapist.

I was still in my job, as my training was on weekends. So, I continued my chats with those who would pull up beside me and we would all feel better. I still enjoyed it. I was in work one day and again I cannot remember how I came across it, but I saw an ad for Indian Head Massage training. It was 2009. I read all about how great it was at helping with stress, anxiety, pain, etc. and thought "Isn't that a wonderful thing! I can help people feel relaxed and happy and pain-free. Happy days!" So I enrolled in that course and qualified as an Indian Head Massage Therapist (IHM). I soon found though that clients would get relief but after a few weeks or maybe a month or two, they would come back with the same problem! Why? Why was this persistently showing up in this person? I am a very curious person. I always ask "But why?" I like to figure out why things do not always work as they should. I find it hard to 'just accept things as they are' without questioning them. It did not take me long to realise that IHM Therapy was NOT going to be what I would do for a living either.

So, I kept on working. I was getting very disillusioned by this stage. "Maybe I should just give up and stay in my job?" It was now 2010 and I had turned forty years of age the previous December. My kids bought me a laptop as a birthday present. (Turned out to be the best gift ever). I was feeling very lost in my life at that time. No idea what I was going to do next. The urge to leave where I worked was getting stronger. But, we had purchased our first home just before the Celtic Tiger period in Ireland ended. The work dried up slowly for my then partner and we were getting into debt. Things were not going well in our relationship and my kid's hated living where we had moved to. It was a tough time for everyone.

I remember browsing the internet on my new laptop and wandering, seemingly aimlessly around the web. I came across something called EFT, which stood for Emotional Freedom Techniques. It was interesting but I did not really get it, so I moved on. But as they say, if something shows up three times in a row, PAY ATTENTION! So, I did. Being curious, I decided to look deeper into this weird little process that promised to do so much so quickly. I was hooked.

That was in January 2010. I was booked on the next training course which started in March of that year. I had no idea how I was going to pay for it, but I just knew I had to do it. I had to trust that if it was right for me that the Universe would provide a way for me to do it. The EFT training was held over three residential weekends at a beautiful house in Tipperary. After three months of training and practice, I was now a Certified EFT Practitioner. This was it. I had found exactly what I was looking for. Applying Tapping while someone is 'Tuned into' in other words, talking about their issue, allows the client to get instant relief from the uncomfortable emotions they are experiencing. They can quickly release the emotions and negative beliefs that were created during the event. Imagine how happy I was about this!

When we release old emotions from our energy system, it allows us to be more connected to our true selves. We can access our Inner Being and Source Energy. One of the things I love about this practice is that once I teach it to my client, they can do it between sessions when they feel they need to. In fact, I often have clients do Tapping homework. I think it is very empowering for them to know that they can take charge of how they feel. That they do not need to wait until the next session to feel better.

During the following year, a family member got sick and I had to take time off work to take care of them. Little did I know that I would be called to use ALL the training that I had done. I used EFT for myself while I was supporting them in getting well. And for the stress I was experiencing when having to deal with banks about our mortgage arrears. I would tap before making calls to the electric company and all the other people I owed money to. I used EFT when I finally decided to leave my partner of twenty-four years and when I had to leave my home. I also deliberately applied the Law of Attraction when I was making calls and when I was looking for a new place to live. I can honestly say that without EFT, I would most definitely not have managed as well as I did emotionally.

So, that is the story of how I came to learn about EFT. It is the one thing I use regularly in my Law of Attraction Coaching Practice. I will give an example of how I use EFT to help clients with beliefs, exam pressure, sports performance and But, just let me say one thing… *You Are Already Enough.*

It is true. Right here, right now, no matter how broken you feel or what problems you have, You Are Enough. This is what I had to keep reminding myself of during those difficult years. I felt so ashamed that I could not pay my mortgage. So overwhelmed and frustrated that I could not provide all the things my kids needed. I just had to keep reminding myself that I was doing the best I knew how.

The first part of the Tapping Process is to create a Set-Up Statement. That statement is "Even though I have this 'issue', I deeply and completely accept myself". For example, I used: "Even though I have this fear in my stomach when I think about making this phone call, I deeply and completely accept myself". This helped me to make the call without feeling the fear. Which helped me to manifest someone who was really helpful.

Accepting ourselves for where we are now and how we are feeling is the key to unlocking your very own healing capabilities.

When we are living with physical pain, grief, fear, anxiety, addiction, guilt, phobias, debt, shame or trauma (personal or group) or any other issues we can sometimes feel less than whole. We feel that we cannot accept ourselves because of what we are experiencing. We may even judge ourselves very harshly. In my experience with clients, it usually comes down to how they were shamed as a child when they were struggling with something. The parents/caregivers did not know how to handle what the child was feeling. So, they would dismiss them in some way. The child would then feel ashamed to express their emotions and would not feel safe to allow them.

As you may know already, unexpressed emotions cause us to experience situations over and over until we allow ourselves to express them. And if they remain unexpressed for a long time, they can cause dis-ease in our body. When we experience situations over and over we create beliefs about them.

An example that comes to mind is a client (I will call him John) who had issues with money. He was good at earning it but never seemed to have enough. Something 'unexpected' would show up so that he would have to spend the extra money that he had earned. So, he could never get ahead. Using EFT during coaching sessions around his money issues, John recalled a memory he had when he was about ten years of age. His mother asked him to go to the shop to get a few groceries. So, he headed off with his father and arrived at the small local shop. John handed the list to the shopkeeper and he went about getting the bits he needed. The shopkeeper convinced John to buy a few other bits (that were not on the shopping list) and he thought it was a great idea to get them as it might cheer his mother up. They got into the car and headed home. When his mother saw what he had bought, she was terribly angry. She shouted at John and told him that he should not have bought the extra items. John felt so ashamed and stupid. He was sent to his room and as you can imagine, he felt so guilty and bad about himself. He discovered that he took on a belief that day, "I'm really bad at handling money." The dis-ease that John had was showing up in his beliefs about money. Money is something that we need in our lives. So, this was not helpful at all. It was causing a lot of stress and feelings of failure and guilt.

Releasing Shame, Guilt And Old Beliefs Using 'Tell The Story' Technique

To release the emotions around the memory that John had about that trip to the shop and how it ended, I used the Tell the Story Technique. He gave the story a name 'The shopping trip'. I asked John to let me know how he would feel IF I asked him to just think about the shopping trip story. He was feeling anxious in his stomach and he rated the anxiety at a 6 out of 10. 10 being the highest intensity. (remember that I am not asking him to tell me the story yet, I'm just asking how he'd feel if I asked him to tell me). We started to tap for the anxiety he felt until it went down to about a 2 in intensity. I asked him if he would feel ok to start telling me about what happened. He was happy to start.

This is why I love this technique; it is so gentle, and it takes away the fear or anxiety about discussing an issue that is highly emotional. Unlike Talk Therapy in which we just dive right in, I asked John to start in a place that felt safe, like being asked to go to the shop for his mother (he was so excited and felt like a 'big boy'). He proceeded with the story and each time he felt a 'spike' in his energy, like feeling fear or anxiety, we would stop and tap. I would ask him to start at the beginning of the story again, stopping each time he felt any emotional intensity. By the end of the story, John had no emotions attached to the memory. He said it was like watching a movie. What John was experiencing was being emotionally free from the experience. He felt sad for his mother; he knew how hard she had worked to earn money for the shopping. He could now see that his mother was angry because she was in fear. She was afraid because she had less money and had probably been hoping to pay for other things. John could now see from an adult perspective, why his mother reacted that way and that it wasn't his fault as he said, "I was only ten years old! No one had ever taught me how to shop!"

He could also see how the belief he took on that day was still playing out in his life. Through releasing the emotions of that memory, he is now free to choose a different belief. His new affirmation is "I am good with money. I am responsible with money and I always have enough". If I had tried to get John to create this affirmation before, it would not have worked. He would not have believed it and therefore, his situation with money would not change. Affirmations DO NOT WORK unless we believe them to be true. The Law of Attraction does NOT hear your words, it responds to your vibration. By finding and clearing the subconscious memory (the TRUE affirmation) there is no conflict between his conscious and subconscious beliefs. So, now he can manifest money more easily and allow himself to hold onto it.

This technique took about one hour to complete. It would have taken many sessions for John to have this cognitive shift in understanding what had happened using Talk Therapy alone.

Think about how you feel about something that is happening for you right now. What thoughts come to your mind about YOU having this issue? Are you judging yourself for being in debt? Being overweight? Being in physical pain for years? Or living with anxiety? When we judge ourselves, we are not practicing self-acceptance. You may have heard the saying attributed to Carl Jung "What we resist persists". Our resistance to acknowledging what we are feeling or what is happening in our lives is preventing us from being free of it.

However, when we acknowledge what we are thinking, feeling, and experiencing, we have now brought it to light. Once we bring it into the light (from the subconscious to the conscious) we can then apply EFT to it and release it. We can understand it and we have the opportunity (with support) to process it and let it go, just like John did with his memory. He resisted all the feelings he had about it like, shame and guilt. When he acknowledged them and

ALLOWED them to be processed, the memory no longer had any power over him.

Basic Premise of EFT: 'The Cause of All Negative Emotions Is A Disruption in The Body's Energy System' Gary Craig. EFT Founder. https://emofree.com/

The negative emotions we feel when we focus on our 'issue' are a direct result of the thoughts we have about it. Because our thoughts are vibrational in nature, they are sent like a signal out to the Universe and we attract more of the thing we were thinking about. Whether what we are thinking about is wanted or unwanted we get more of that. When John got to a point in his finances where he felt like he was 'getting ahead', he would ultimately sabotage his success by creating an experience where he had to get rid of the 'extra' money. Doing this would prove him right. He was 'bad at handling money' that he could 'never get ahead'. And so, the cycle would continue. Human beings love being right. So, when we prove to ourselves that we are 'right' we feel better. "See I told you. I was right!" But would you rather be right than happy?

I'd like to give you a few examples of how I've used EFT for other issues.

Exam Fears

I used EFT to help a friend's daughter who was really struggling with her maths at school. She was about to do her Leaving Certificate and was so afraid that she would fail the maths exam which she really needed to pass. We tapped for an hour or so, on all the feelings she had about maths and her upcoming exam. I met her a few months later and I had forgotten that we had done the session. I asked her how she got on with the exam. She replied "Yeah, I was grand. I was not a bit nervous at all. It was great!" And of course, she passed. She is now a nurse and loves her job.

Sport Performance Issues

When I had just qualified as an EFT Practitioner, a friend at work asked me if EFT would help with sport performance issues. She was the captain of the local camogie team and they had not won the County Finals for the last two years. She asked if I would come along to do some Tapping with the team. I told her that I would be delighted to take them through a session. I was so nervous! This was my first group session and I had to stand in front of them and explain this weird little technique and how tapping on their face and torso may help them win the County Finals! I tapped on my own fears before I went in and I was fine. I had them get into smaller groups. I gave them all pens and paper and asked them to write down their doubts and fears around playing in the Finals.

This exercise was immensely powerful. There were tears as they bonded with each other through their fears. They had no idea that their team members felt just as much fear and anxiety as they did. Each had their own individual reasons for the fear, but they all had fear. I took the sheets of paper and we started to Tap on all the issues they had listed. I showed the list to their two coaches who were sitting at the back of the room. I said to them "Look how much energy that is being spent on dealing with these fears. Once they remove them, they will be able to think more clearly and make better decisions on the pitch". I had no idea how it was going to turn out. BUT, they went on to win the County Finals that year. Did EFT help? My guess is yes it did. The captain thought so too and mentioned me in her speech after they won. It was great fun to do and it just shows the power of a group Tapping session.

What is EFT?

EFT is a Somatic, Cognitive, Energetic Practice. Created by Gary Craig in 1995 based on his understanding of Dr Roger Callaghan's work in TFT (Thought Field Therapy) Here's a great little video that will give you an idea of who EFT works https://www.youtube.com/watch?v=VFKVVP8KXd4&t=21s

Somatic: The sensation or emotion we have in our body when we are experiencing or remembering an 'issue'. The other somatic part being that we tap on our physical body with our fingertips.

Cognitive: Meaning, we use words (to describe the issue at hand and how we feel about it) as we do in Talk Therapy to identify the issue. We use EFT to bypass the conscious mind, which helps us find subconscious beliefs, etc.

Energetic: Meridians are pathways in the body that carry energy or Chi as the Chinese call it. These pathways can get blocked due to stress and trauma, which results in a disruption in the energy system, this disruption, if not dealt with, can cause dis-ease or illness. Tapping gently on the meridian end points addresses the disruption and brings the body back into balance.

The good thing is you do not have to have any knowledge of the Meridian System for EFT to work for you.

EFT stands for Emotional Freedom Techniques and is not to be confused with the Tapping you may see online. The words 'Techniques' should be a clue... We use several powerful techniques in our sessions. I gave you an example of one of them earlier. The technique we use will depend on the intensity the client experiences during a session. The main priority in all sessions is to prevent the client from being re–traumatised.

Unfortunately, not all practitioners are aware that this can happen and may not be trained well in using the techniques. This can cause the client to believe that EFT is making them worse!

There is no doubt that you will feel uncomfortable when you are addressing whatever issue you have. We must allow ourselves to look at and feel the emotion of what we experienced to be free of it. BUT using the techniques like Tell the Story or Tearless Trauma, you can move quickly through the emotions attached to the memory and set yourself free. Therefore, we call it Emotional FREEDOM Techniques.

YouTube is full of Tapping Videos. There are thousands of Tapping Scripts. The problem with these are that many people tap along to the video or use the Tapping Script, get some relief, feel great for a while and then the symptoms or issue shows up again. They then believe that EFT does not work! What has really happened is, they have successfully let go of some energy around the 'issue', i.e. got some temporary relief, but they did not get ALL the aspects of the issue dealt with.

Whenever we experience something traumatic, our mind captures all parts of that event and stores it as a memory. The sounds, sights, smells, time of day, what people were present etc. It takes a snapshot, so to speak. It then files it away. When we find ourselves in a situation that resembles that traumatic event, our mind will automatically recall the previous trauma, it will pull up that file and remind you about what happened. It does that by sending signals to you via our feelings, which causes us to go into Fight, Flight or Freeze mode. Our minds only job is to protect us at all costs.

For example, if you had an experience in school where you had to read out loud in front of the class and you made a mistake, then the other kids starting sniggering or the teacher made you feel stupid, this may play out in your adult life when you're asked to give a presentation at work. Your mind reminds you that it is not safe to do this. And so, your palms start sweating, and your mouth goes dry, you want the ground to open and swallow you.

(This can be challenging when you want to do something new, it can 'over-protect you', causing you to play it safe and stay right where you are). Try tapping on old memories like these. Or find a Practitioner that you feel comfortable working with.

To find out how to use it for pain relief, you can watch me take two people through the Tapping Process. You can tap along yourself if you have any pain. Pain is the body's way of letting us know that we have emotions that need to be released. It is worth a try! Go Here: https://youtu.be/n_QwnuSaym8

I was in my forties when I awakened to my potential. Your potential is only as limited as you believe it to be. It is never too late to do something different with your life. If you really love something and it comes easy to you, there is a reason for that. Do not let your fears hold you back. Lean into them. Tap on those fears! Do not give up on finding that one thing that brings it all together for you. I am glad I did not give up. I just kept asking why. I was always given the answer. You are too. You just must listen and take that first step.

Remember who you really are. You are an amazing being and you can use your mind to deliberately create your life. We have beliefs that have been inherited and beliefs that we created through our own life experiences. Either way, we need to take responsibility for what we are creating and decide to let go of the beliefs and family paradigms that no longer serve us. We can choose to do this not only for ourselves but for our children. For just as you inherited your beliefs from your family, so will they inherit yours. Beliefs are energy patterns and they can be transformed. It is up to each one of us to be brave enough to look at them and decide what to do with them. EFT can help you do that. Look at your beliefs with curiosity and an open mind.

My Current Work

I went on to become a Certified Law of Attraction Coach & Creating Money Coach in 2015 with Christy Whitman at the Quantum Success Coaching Academy. I now teach other coaches and healers how to rapidly create more money and a thriving practice without working harder or longer. I do this using proven Law of Attraction techniques and processes. EFT features heavily in my One to One Mentorship Program and my Radical Money Mindset Signature Club.

Find out more here www.radicalmoneymindset.com

Feel free to join me on my Facebook Business Page for more on EFT & Law of Attraction.

https://www.facebook.com/RadicalMoneyMindset

When you get used to using EFT for yourself, you can absolutely use it on any issue. I do highly recommend that you seek the guidance of a qualified practitioner when working on bigger issues. EFT works well alongside other therapies. Please advise your therapist or doctor if you choose to use EFT while under their care.

Reclaim Your Fertility
by Denise Christie

Twenty years ago, it would not have entered my head to become a fertility coach. In fact, during my years of working as a busy legal executive, I would have scoffed at the thoughts of using any complementary or alternative therapy as a treatment for anything. After years of legal training and working for solicitors, my thinking had become very black and white and there was no woolly middle thinking that would have allowed the notion that anything other than prescribed medicine could fix any health issues I might face. However, all that was to change when my experiences of multiple miscarriages led me firmly down the holistic path.

My first pregnancy was textbook perfect. I do not recall ever feeling so vibrant, energised, and healthy. It was also probably one of the happiest times of my life. Two of my friends were pregnant at the same time and they could not work out how I was having such an easy time of it while they suffered through morning sickness, lack of energy and mood swings.

However, the labour was a totally different kettle of fish. In fact, it was a traumatic and frightening experience. It started off so well. I was completely laid back when I went into labour. I went to bingo with my husband because I was so bored at home. We were very chilled and did not really rush to the hospital until we felt we needed to go. However, things did not progress well and after thirty-nine hours of labouring, my daughter had managed to get herself well and truly wedged. I caught a concerned glance between the midwife and the nurse.

Seconds later, the doors of the delivery suite swung open, the ambient lighting was swapped for full-on fluorescents and half a dozen medics rushed in – all determined to deliver this baby! Within thirty minutes, Alice was finally born. I remember the medical team forming a wall of bodies to my left and behind my husband.

Had I not been totally exhausted at that stage, I might have been more aware of what was going on and been more concerned, but the truth was I didn't find out until days later when I was reading my discharge notes that my daughter had been born not breathing and had to be resuscitated. No one had told me. Perhaps they assumed I knew, but that was the first of many incidences of non-medical disclosure.

We took our gorgeous little daughter home and within a short period of time and being fully occupied with the raising our daughter, the trauma of the birth was soon forgotten.

I had already decided to take an extended maternity leave at this stage. The law firm I worked for had an amazing maternity package and I had worked up until three days before Alice was born which meant I could carry over the extra weeks I had worked on to the end of my maternity time.

A few months before I was due to return to work, my husband and I talked about trying for a second. It made perfect sense! We had it all worked out that if we got pregnant straight away, I would only have to return to work for four months before I would be leaving again for my next maternity leave. It would also mean that our little family would be complete as we did not want any more than two children

I had fallen pregnant with Alice straight away – I just knew instinctively it would happen the same way again. My husband

and I used to joke about passing each other in the bathroom – that is how quick I could get pregnant. Sure enough, within weeks of deciding to have a second child, I was pregnant.

When we were pregnant with Alice, we told people almost as soon as we found out. We were so excited and just could not wait to spread the news. This time we decided to keep it to ourselves – partly because we thought there might be questions and worries from family about getting pregnant again so soon and managing two small children.

When I miscarried at eight weeks, we were so glad we never told anyone. It was hard enough to deal with the loss, but having to tell our friends and family about it would have made it even harder.

My second miscarriage was eight days before my return to work from maternity leave. I remember like it was yesterday, sitting back at my desk and asking people not to come near me because I was struggling to contain my emotions. Luckily, I had a little booth all to myself, so I could avoid others if I wanted to. They assumed I was tearful because I missed Alice, and of course, a large part of my sadness was because I had left her for the first time since she was born. I loved my job, had a great boss and what should have been a happy time of being back with friends and colleagues, was torture. Nobody had even known we were pregnant; how could I tell them what else was breaking my heart?

After the third miscarriage, my doctor was finally ready to have a conversation other than, "It's perfectly normal." "It happens to more couples than you realise." "You're young you can try again", and "Why don't you concentrate on your lovely daughter for now!" I had some blood tests that all came back totally normal. There seemed to be no reason for the miscarriages. She told me to relax!

By the time we had our fifth miscarriage, we were starting to hit the rocks in our relationship. Neither of us was coping particularly well. I was over-emotional, and I saw my husband's lack of emotion as a void of empathy towards me.

It was around this time that we discovered my medical history. But only by badgering my GP non-stop to send me for an appointment with a gynaecologist. It turned out there had been some damage done internally because of the delay in delivering Alice. She had gotten stuck in the birth canal and this was why she was born not breathing.

This knowledge raised more questions than it answered. I was left wondering if there had been medical intervention earlier, could that have been avoided. Alice and I have a little private joke between us now – usually around her birthday – when I remind her that she broke my vagina!!

By the time we had the eighth miscarriage, we were utterly broken as a couple, and I was literally on the point of a breakdown. When the inevitable happened and my husband and I separated, I was left juggling my legal work, the sale of our beloved home and the search for somewhere new for me and my daughter to live.

After one particularly scary day when I felt tempted to step off the pavement into the path of a London black cab, I realised it was time to get help. I was referred to a counsellor by my GP. I cannot even remember the type of therapy I was getting – all I remember is stepping into her office and crying from the moment I arrived to the moment I left, every single time I had an appointment with her.

A friend of mine suggested I try aromatherapy which I initially considered a ridiculous suggestion, so I was naturally hugely sceptical. When you work in the field of law, you develop very black and white thinking. Nowhere in that thinking could I find room for the notion that rubbing smelly oils on to my skin could fix what was going on in my head.

However, after about three months of regular treatments, I remember walking out of the treatment room and into the fresh air and this thought just popped into my head "I want my clients to feel this way". To this day, I have no idea where that thought came from, but it was the catalyst for a massive change in career.

I had worked hard for years to study for my legal executive qualifications and loved my job. Then out of the blue, my boss announced he was taking early retirement. Another blow! I had worked for him for nearly fourteen years and he had coached and supported me through my training and career. So, even though I was offered another more senior position in the firm when the time came, I decided to take redundancy and listen to that voice I had heard so clearly that day about having my own clients. There began my journey into holistic medicine. I started a two-year full-time course in holistic at Canterbury College later that year.

There is no doubt it all seemed 'woo woo' at times, but I suppose by the time I started college, I had seen the results for myself. And that was a massive leap for me, having worked in law for so long.

Almost two years later and shortly after qualifying, I picked up a buy and sell type newspaper, I had never looked through before. The paper opened on the houses and land section and, there in front of me was a picture of a little cottage and I immediately fell in love with it. Whatever possessed me, I contacted the owner to make enquiries about buying it. I loved it even more once I saw the pictures that she emailed to me.

There was only one problem. The house was in Galway in the West of Ireland, and I lived in Kent in the East of England. I flew out to see the house and had the most amazing experienced when I walked up the path. I felt as though I had always lived there. The day after flying back, I put my house on the market, made an offer on the house in Ireland and a little over eight weeks later – the deal was done!!

Immediately, I set about building up a holistic practice. My first treatment room was above a health store, then I moved it to a spare room in my home because of difficulties with childminders and then eventually put up a purpose-built treatment cabin in the field behind the house.

As had happened so many times before, another catalyst for change and growth then came into my life. This time in the shape of a client, I had known for quite a while. She arrived for her treatment one day and she was booked to have a massage. She then told me she was six weeks pregnant. I was thrilled for her and started to discuss with her some different treatment options as I was reluctant to do a massage on someone who was only six weeks pregnant. And then she began to cry. I was so confused. I could not work out why she would be crying. When she told me, this was not her first pregnancy and said how many miscarriages she had gone through. I felt the room spin as the air was being pulled from my lungs. I recognised her grief and despair. Like me, no-one other than her husband knew of their many losses. And she pleaded with me to help her find a way to hold on to this baby.

I set about creating a treatment plan for her and pulled in everything I knew about cellular memory, about affirmations, about creating a different DNA. Everything we now know about the science of epigenetics. I saw her every week for her treatment and checked in with her mindset regularly. There was a certain medical definition she had been given and I had asked her never to say it or think it again. On the 34th week of her pregnancy, her husband brought her to me for a final treatment en route to the hospital for an elected c-section and she gave birth to a perfectly healthy baby boy. I will always think of her son as the very first Health and Harmony baby!

At that point, my practical brain kicked back in. I realised I needed to have a deeper understanding of treatments that would help other women like her. There was extraordinarily little out there at the time, and of course, some 'Mickey Mouse' courses as there always are. So, I set about researching what treatments would help support women in holding on to their pregnancies and to help them get pregnant in the first place as I was starting to see many women in my clinic who were experiencing problems with fertility.

I decided to only train with who I considered the best in the field of fertility. Over the years, I have now added fertility massage, fertility acupuncture, mindfulness, health coaching and fertility counselling to my toolkit. I currently work primarily as a fertility coach and therapist from my treatment room outside of Loughrea in Galway, specialising in supporting couples trying to conceive and those struggling to remain pregnant.

As a one-time sceptic of holistic medicine, myself, today I enjoy being asked if there is any evidence to back up the way I practice. I am always itching to demonstrate the research. Although my methods when as a complete system may appear 'woo woo', when you break each element down, there is scientific proof to back up the effectiveness of every layer.

The first layer is getting to grips with changing the message you send your body – so basically it the science of epigenetics. The next layer is nutrition, with plenty of scientific research into the benefits of both macronutrients and micronutrients.

Unfortunately, miscarriage and infertility are still massively taboo subjects in Ireland. I have worked with clients who have not even told their parents, siblings, or best friends they are struggling. But of course, I understand that position, given my personal experience.

We are brought up to believe we are innately fertile. We spent our teenage years and most of our twenties in fear of getting pregnant. But the emotions wrapped into a struggle are around shame and failure, and for guys can go even deeper than that – affecting the core of their masculinity.

As a result of my current knowledge and training, I now believe that my struggles with miscarriage stemmed from a combination of factors: from physical damage sustained during my daughter's birth, a highly stressful job, undiagnosed coeliac disease and my 'hatred' towards my body for failing me.

A favourite expression of mine is "You don't know what you don't know". Twenty years ago, there were a lot of things I did not know. I did not have a clue how to manage out of control stress levels or that a twelve hour working day was not supporting my yearning to have more children. I did not know how to listen to my body instead of giving out to her all the time, nor was I aware of the devastating effect all that negative self-talk was having on my fertility. I did not know that what little food I was eating had nothing nutritionally valuable to offer a body trying desperately hard to hold on to a pregnancy. And I did not understand the importance of focusing on my relationship with my husband ABOVE ALL ELSE!

I did not know these things twenty years ago ... but today I do. I did not know them in time to help me through my struggle to build my family. But I do know them now. And it is this knowledge, together with the specific training I have gone through, that enable me to help so many couples who are stuck in a struggle to conceive or a struggle to hold on to their pregnancy.

In the back of my mind, there is always a realisation that if I had met someone with my skillset twenty years ago, my story could have been quite different. Of course, that makes me sad when I think of my daughter being an only child and that I could not give her a brother or a sister. But I do try not to dwell on that. Instead, I focus on the positive from my experience, which is, without having gone through my struggle, I would more than likely never be working to help couples overcome their fertility struggle.

Since setting up my practice, Health and Harmony, I have worked with dozens of couples, and at the point of writing this chapter fifty-six babies have been born with four more are "on the way".

I simply cannot describe the joy I experience, from the moment I receive a message or a phone call to tell me they are pregnant, and then most couples will message me when their baby is born. I feel elated for days after.

A struggle to get pregnant is becoming increasingly common. Today, as many as one in six couples are still trying to get pregnant a year after they started trying. A further one in eight couples have still not achieved a pregnancy after two years of trying.

That is a dramatic difference to fertility rates thirty years ago and what is more worrying is that studies show that infertility is expected to increase in the future.

So, what has changed? The truth is plenty has changed! Thirty years ago, the average age that women had their first child was around twenty-one years of age. Today, that age is closer to twenty-seven or twenty-eight and for many women that starting point is in their thirties.

Many couples are waiting longer to start their families – they may want to finish their educations first, or get established in their careers, or be living in the right house for raising their family.

Divorce and remarriage are also much more common– impacting the fertility window. The truth is – female fertility starts to decrease from the age of thirty-five. When you think about it, the older you are, the more likely you are to be exposed to environmental toxins and more likely to be taking medication for health problems.

As well as medical factors, several other issues could be to blame, such as poor nutrition and increased stress levels. With so many factors to take into account, it is clear no single solution is likely to resolve the problem.

The practice of Traditional Chinese Medicine holds the belief that the health and wellbeing of both parents at the time of and/or three months before conception are key to the health of the child conceived.

I have named the fertility programme I created 'Reclaim Your Fertility' mainly because I believe in most cases, we can regain complete control over our ability to become pregnant, once we take responsibility for that.

Of course, every couple is different, but my approach has been to work on what I view are the five main pillars that form the very foundation of your fertility. An imbalance even in one of these can affect your ability to get pregnant.

Most people would believe that parenthood begins the moment a baby exits the mother's womb. I believe that you become a parent; the very moment you decide to create a baby. What is compelling about this is that it empowers each couple to do everything in their power to create a happy, healthy pregnancy and naturally concludes in a happy, healthy baby.

The pillars I ask my couples to concentrate on are:

- Nutrition
- Your relationship
- Stress levels
- Lifestyle
- Your message

Pillar 1 – Nutrition

Nutrition is the first key to fertility and is a fundamental concept in Traditional Chinese Medicine also. Think of it as preparing the soil for planting your garden seeds. If the soil is poor quality and has not received essential nutrients and adequate hydration, if you have not removed the stones and the weeds, the seeds are unlikely to grow and flourish.

When it comes to eating healthily, however, what you are putting in your mouth is only half of the equation. The other half is HOW you eat! What you eat, when you eat and even the mood you are in when you are eating are all crucial elements to consider when it comes to nutrition. Slowing down at mealtimes, paying attention to the food you are eating and savouring every single bite all allow your digestive system to do the job it was perfectly designed to do.

Also, exposure to chemicals such as fertilisers and pesticides is also something to consider as an overload of these can interfere with fertility hormones.

Your body is the best, most efficient experimental laboratory to determine the effect that food has on you.

Have you ever eaten a takeaway or a 'builder's breakfast' and spent the next few hours feeling lethargic, queasy, and questioning the wisdom of what you just ate?

That is your body giving you that message – and it did not cost you a cent to find out that what you ate was not healthy for you.

Aim to keep your food 'clean and green' as much as you are able. Eat organic where you can. The body's digestive system was never designed to deal with the amount of chemical exposure currently present in our food. Reducing your exposure to highly processed foods and those foods which have been exposed to harmful chemicals will help keep you away from the GP.

Get used to thinking of food in terms of its function. For instance, protein helps with egg and sperm formation; carbohydrates provide energy for the body to perform essential functions, greens are for cleaning and mopping up the nasties. These are all essential components and it is good to have a healthy mix of all three.

Get in the habit of reading labels on your food. If you cannot pronounce some of the ingredients, they should not be in your shopping trolley. As a rule of thumb 'whole foods' contain no more than four or five ingredients. If the ingredient list is any longer than that, pop it back on the shelf. It is not food — it has just been carefully crafted to look like food!

When to supplement. As a rule of thumb, I will always recommend supplementing to fill any potential gaps in your nutrition. As your nutrition improves, you can start to pull back on the amount or how frequently you take them.

Pillar 2 – Your Relationship

Any persistent struggle can affect even the strongest of relationships. A struggle to get pregnant adds in another layer because the potential answer to that struggle involves making love! Once you add strong emotions such as anger, guilt fear and performance anxiety into that mix, then you may have a problem! Because who wants to make love when they are angry with their partner?

If you are struggling to conceive, it can become extremely easy to consider lovemaking to be a 'chore' rather than the wonderful experience it once was. This is especially true if you are undergoing any form of fertility treatment. The irony is that the more fizz there is in your lovemaking, the more likely you are to conceive. The good news is, it is easier than you think to put the fizz back into your love life.

As human beings, we are naturally tactile creatures – which is why we enjoy holding hands, hugging, rubbing our feet off each other etc. Physical contact releases endorphins, the body's natural 'feel-good' factor. Cuddling also releases oxytocin which, as well as creating a sense of wellbeing and joy, can also help you to conceive.

Problems with fertility create an underlying level of stress which can start to permeate every area of your life and raised stress levels create havoc with your hormonal balance. Suddenly, every newspaper article or TV programme appears to feature someone who has become effortlessly pregnant. It can be natural for couples to bottle up their feelings – possibly because they are in denial or it could be, and they do not want to hurt their partner's feelings. This can quite quickly end up causing a rift between the couple. Your partner is the person you are hoping to be raising a child with, they are the person you trust most with your innermost feelings and fears – so naturally, they are the person most able to offer you the support you need. This is a journey you are on together, so it is important to share your fears and your worries.

All the opinions and discussions you had before you both decided to have a baby together are just as important as they ever were. These are the things that connected you both when you first met and the ground on which your relationship grew and thrived. Steer your focus away from the fertility conversations whenever you can to keep the connection between you strong.

At times it will be the last thing on your mind- but finding and hanging on to your sense of humour can be one of the best things you can do to prevent becoming overshadowed by your fertility journey. Laughter is one of the most powerful antidotes to stress. It lightens your burdens and keeps you grounded and hopeful. Watch a funny film, go to a comedy show, share funny stories – and benefit from all those lovely mood-enhancing endorphins.

There is no more effective way to let your partner know they are important to you than by booking a night out together. An evening in a restaurant, at the cinema or bowling alley give you both the opportunity to reconnect and make each other a priority. Make sure the date is in the calendar and cannot be cancelled. Use the evening as an opportunity to reconnect and re-learn why you love this person and what they mean to you.

Sprucing up the bedroom and making it an inviting and intimate place works wonders for your love life. Free the bedroom of any clutter and soften the lighting. Add in some candles and romantic music and hey presto, you have turned your bedroom into a bona fide love nest!

One thing I advise every couple to do, even if it is for a couple of months, is to stop tracking her cycle. It is tempting to become obsessed with your fertile days. If this happens, there is a possibility that you are only making love on the days, you consider yourself to be fertile. This can have a detrimental effect for two reasons.

Firstly, it can have a damaging effect on your partner's ability to achieve or maintain an erection. On top of that, your partner may also feel you only want to make love on your fertile days, reducing his role in the baby-making process to that of sperm donor. If making love shifts from being a tender act of connection and pleasure to being a necessity, that can play havoc with a man's emotions and in turn, negatively affect his ability to perform.

Making love is often discouraged for couples who cannot get pregnant without assisted fertility. If you are a couple who, for whatever reason, cannot get pregnant without some form of assisted fertility, a recommendation to stop making love can potentially decrease your chances of getting pregnant. The strength of a relationship, the struggle of fertility and the stress attached to that all play a potential role in male factor infertility.

Pillar 3 – Stress Levels

Medical evidence is mounting of a link between stress and infertility, both as a cause of infertility but also an effect of the anxiety caused by the failure to conceive.

Stress affects the body in many negative ways. In women, the chemical changes that occur can not only affect the cycle but also prevent the maturation and release of the egg. For the guys, it can lead to erectile dysfunction and have an adverse effect on sperm count and motility.

In addition, failure to conceive a desperately longed-for child, repeated medical tests and procedures, and the failure to get to the root of the problem can create a stressful environment. The entire process can become a vicious circle of disappointment and anxiety.

While managing stress does not in itself guarantee a successful fertility outcome, there is compelling evidence that it can help.

There are some essential things you need to know about stress. Firstly, all disease is inflammation. Secondly, stress creates inflammation. And thirdly, you can have the best diet on the planet, but if you are under stress, you are still creating imbalance – because stress trumps food every single time!

A simple breathing meditation that you can take anywhere with you and use at any time can be an invaluable tool to overcoming the effects of stress. It is called the 16-second breath. While counting the numbers in your head, you breathe in for four, hold for four, breathe out for four, then hold the out-breath for four.

Meditation is an effective tool for switching off the stress response. In fact, just twenty minutes of meditation every single day can help to overcome 10-14 hours of daily stress. This simple method of relaxation is the most effective daily tool you can use to dial back the harmful effects of stress. Apps such as Calm,

Buddify or Headspace make it easy to choose a daily meditation, or you can search for specific meditations on the internet. Check out Sharon Fitzmaurice Holistic Wellness on YouTube for free guided meditations.

A simple way to manage stress is to figure out what you can control. Stress is caused by situations that are out of your control. Even if this is the case, there is always something that you can do that is within your control. For example, you cannot control whether your body will release an egg each month, but you can take actions to ensure that when an egg is released that it will be the healthiest version that egg can be!

Pillar 4 – Lifestyle

In modern-day society, there are so many lifestyle factors that can potentially affect your ability to conceive. Long working hours, shift work, a long commute to work, allowing time to eat at work, family commitments, environmental exposure at work, toxic work environments, leaving little or no time for relaxation or healthy exercise .... - the list is potentially endless! Of course, not all these factors can be changed – but what you can change is how you manage the effects that they have on your fertility health.

Moving your body enhances your fertility. Movement creates healthy blood flow to enrich the reproductive region and nourish the womb, eggs, and sperm. Moving the body also releases feel-good hormones which help to override the effects of stress and reduce inflammation.

The important thing is to find a movement that works for you – yoga, swimming, walking, jogging. We are not all cut out for the gym, but our body loves some form of movement. It increases the blood supply, bringing oxygen and nutrients and speeds up the circulation of the lymph. A healthy lymph system is crucial for a healthy immune system.

Pillar 5 – Your Message

Every time you have a thought, the food choices you make, the social and physical environment you live in — can all affect your DNA. It is a theory backed up by the science of epigenetics.

Hearing a diagnosis that may leave a lasting impression can create a belief that it will always be the case. For instance, hearing that you are 'infertile' could make you believe that you will ALWAYS be infertile.

So, if your DNA is negatively influenced by poor choices — the good news is you can totally reverse that by making better, healthier choices! One of the most important things you can do very easily is changing the conversation you are having with yourself every single day.

Sit quietly and discover your current inner message. For some who have been struggling to conceive that message can be quite negative. 'I can't get pregnant.' 'There must be something wrong with me.' 'My womb does not work.'

What would you like that message to be? 'I am fabulously fertile.' 'My womb is perfect.' 'I am happy and healthy.'

Those messages might seem alien at first, especially if you are in the habit of repeating a negative message to yourself. But the fact is, the message you are currently giving yourself is not necessarily the truth either!

By changing the message, you are re-coding the computer. Creating a healthier, more positive message, alongside taking steps to improve other areas of your lifestyle, and eating habits which are potentially affecting your fertility can combine to create a fabulously fertile version of you!

Every thought you think, every word you say is an 'affirmation.' From our childhood, we develop thought patterns and belief systems and every affirmation we think or say reflects these thoughts or beliefs. Every time you say or believe or think something negative about your body or your health – you perpetuate that situation.

The good news is you can use positive affirmations to challenge negative beliefs and to replace them with positive self-nurturing beliefs. It is a kind of 'brainwashing' only you get to choose which negative beliefs to wash away. The more determined you are to make your changes, the better they will work for you. Continually repeating affirmations with conviction will chip away at even the strongest resistance. Changing the way you think, reprogramming your mind and removing the old negative beliefs can enable you to achieve the life, health, and fertility you have always wanted for yourself.

Success Stories

One of my clients came to me two weeks before her third round of IVF. I told her that there was little I could do to influence that round as we had too little time, but that I would try and do what I could to support her. Unfortunately, that round was not successful.

When she had had time to recover emotionally from that setback, she came back to me again and we started working together on a regular basis for three months before she went abroad for her next retrieval and transfer.

My focus during that time was on improving the health and vitality of her womb lining and the quality of her eggs. I also worked with her husband to show him changes he could make to improve the quality of his sperm. This time she conceived twins!

She returned to me again sometime later, having gone through another round of failed IVF in the interim. She had realised the only time the IVF had worked was when we had been working together. So, we started working together again and on her next round of IVF, she conceived another set of twins!

The next time I saw her, the second twins were ten months old. They were all boys, and she was desperate for a girl. But the woman I met this time was not the woman I remembered. She was two stone underweight because she could barely hold down food, had lost a substantial amount of hair, her skin was in dreadful condition, she had absolutely no energy and she had not had a proper menstrual cycle since the birth of the youngest twins.

Her health had been destroyed by the repeated rounds of IVF. She was also feeling depressed because she had a young family that needed her energy and her focus, and a wonderful husband she felt she was neglecting because she had no energy left for him.

We worked together for four months, but I stressed concerns about her getting pregnant until her health returned, so my focus was on getting her sparkle back. In time, she regained her lost weight, her hair grew back, and her energy returned.

When she felt she had got her old self back, she stopped coming, and I did not hear from her for a while. Then one day she called me, out of the blue. She was just out of her doctor's surgery because she had never settled back into a regular cycle and was concerned that she might be having an early menopause, which can often happen after several rounds of IVF. In fact, it was the opposite – she was pregnant! Twenty weeks. And I was the first person she told after her husband. She had another boy!!

Do not get me wrong – I am certainly not against assisted fertility. I have worked with many couples whose only option was to use IVF and we worked to radically improve the success of those treatments. But many years, a small fortune and as we have seen, health, energy, and general wellbeing – can be sacrificed to IVF.

And I have seen too many couples who have spent thousands of euros on it, with nothing to show, and even worse, have sacrificed so much that is good in their lives, including their health for the hope it offers. One couple I worked with had spent €17,000 on IVF before getting pregnant naturally.

Another couple I worked with had undergone two rounds of IUI and a round of IVF before they came to me. They were on the verge of spending £12,000 with a UK clinic who was offering a special '3 for the price of 2' deal on IVF rounds.

I asked them to try natural methods for a while and put the IVF on the back burner. They were reluctant, convinced that IVF was their only option, but eventually, they agreed. The woman was seeing me for a while, then started missing the occasional appointment, then more and more of them. When she did come in, I would go through my standard checklist with her.

Are you managing your stress?

NOPE.

How is your nutrition?

APPALLING!

Are you being diligent about your self-care?

Er ..nah!

I decided tough love was required at this time and pointed out that if she were going through IVF, she would be expected to follow the proper protocol – attend all her appointments, taking daily injections and all sorts of noxious medications which trick the body into thinking it's in a fertile state.

If she missed appointments with the consultant or turned up and shrugged her shoulders when he asked if she were taking her medication, he would fire her! Well, refuse to work with her anyway unless she started following protocol. I told her it was the same with me. My methods work – but only if you work them. I cannot do it for you. You are either serious, or you are not.

When she left that day, angry and upset, I was certain I would never see her again.

Ten days later, she called to make an appointment. She never missed an appointment after that, and she was determinedly doing everything I asked of her. Last year I got the call from her. I had been desperate to receive. She was pregnant! Without IUI, without IVF, without any horrible drugs or intrusive and painful medical procedures. We both cried because we both knew the journey she had taken to get to this point.

And some couples have been given an exceptionally low chance of getting pregnant. In fact, one couple I worked with was told they had a ZERO chance of conceiving naturally. So, they had planned to have IVF and had decided that they were not in a financial position to have repeated rounds of IVF so had decided if that round did not work they would have lost their chances of becoming pregnant. They were referred on to me by a couple I had worked with previously and when we first spoke, they were extremely nervous about working with me and this happens a lot. What I offer is not for everyone, and I get that.

I explained how my methods were likely to radically improve the chances of success of the IVF, so they agreed to give it a go. I worked with both for three months and knew the dates they were planning to go for IVF, which was about two months after they finished working with me. When the time came that I thought would be about the time they would be testing for pregnancy, I called her and got the surprise of my life ...

She told me she was just out of the doctors who had just confirmed she was pregnant. I was so thrilled for her and what came next out of the conversation had me in tears! Because she told me that they had not needed to go for any IVF treatments – that she was pregnant NATURALLY! So not only had they the greatest gift on the planet and the one thing they so desperately wanted, they also had about €6,000 euro sitting in the bank which they had not had to spend on IVF!

So, this couple who had been told had ZERO chance of getting pregnant naturally defied all the odds!! This couple made every change I asked them to make – they lived and breathed fertility wellness! Because it is all about getting your body back to the state that nature intended–the one for whom pregnancy and birth are natural and holistic. But it only works if YOU do the work–just like this couple did.

I cannot wave a magic wand and believe me, there are many times I wish that I could!

Do not get me wrong–I am certainly not against assisted fertility. I have worked with many couples whose only option was to use IVF and we worked to radically improve the success of those treatments. But many years, a small fortune and as we have seen, health, energy, and general wellbeing–can be sacrificed to IVF.

And I have seen too many couples who have spent thousands of euros on it, with nothing to show, and even worse, have sacrificed so much that is good in their lives, including their health for the hope it offers. One couple I worked with had spent €17,000 on IVF before getting pregnant naturally.

Some of the tools in the toolkit I give my clients are far less tangible than changing your diet or managing your stress but certainly no less important when it comes to female wellness! They are all about creating a loving, nurturing relationship with your womb.

One couple I worked with had suffered multiple miscarriages and was left feeling traumatised from the experience and literally hated her womb for not holding on to her babies!

In Chinese Medicine, there is a Meridian or energy line called the 'Bao Mai', This energetic channel links the heart to the womb and allows these two organs to communicate with each other. Imagine it like a dual carriageway with energy flowing in each direction. The energy along this channel must be open and flowing for healthy menstruation and conception to occur.

During a fertility struggle or after suffering one or more miscarriages, this heart—womb connection can become damaged or broken, allowing negative emotions and traumas to become stored in the womb. There are strong and damaging emotions connected with that such as frustration, anger, and fear.

The womb literally becomes an emotional dumping group for all those harmful and hurtful words or, worse still, that you create a total disconnect with your womb – so you are not even acknowledging her very presence.

By sending love and nurturing thoughts to your womb, it is possible to reopen that loving flow, rekindle the connection and heal emotional or physical issues.

The work that this particular couple and I did together was helping her to heal her relationship with her womb and then when she became pregnant four months later, we continued to work together well into her pregnancy until she felt reassured and confident enough to trust that her womb would carry her baby to full term. She gave birth to a beautiful baby girl.

Conclusion

The causes of infertility can be many and varied – they could be related to structural abnormalities, hormonal imbalances, nutritional deficiencies, or many other reasons. Fortunately, you can take back control! There are viable, safe, and effective natural options to not only support and boost your natural fertility but which can also assist with the medical options.

By making changes to your health and lifestyle, you will feel empowered and back in control. And the fabulous news is these changes will not only help you get pregnant but will help you have a healthy baby and a healthy life!

Taking responsibility for your fertility is not about your diagnosis or what is wrong. It is about seeing yourself and a fabulously fertile baby-making machine, seeing yourself as whole and making whatever changes you need to make – while you wait for your baby to arrive!

Imagine if you could change what you eat, say, do and think to recreate a much healthier, much more fertile version of yourself? Think of the possibilities in that? It could mean the end of your struggle to get pregnant. It could bring about the family you have always longed for. It could mean NO MORE expensive, painful, or intrusive medical procedures. Imagine that!

Close your eyes and visualise your heart's desire. What does it look like? What does it feel like? What do you have to do to make it come true? To bring your dream closer to fruition, you need to turn your dreams into goals. List them – be extremely specific. To achieve your goals, you then need to break them down into small, regular, achievable choices.

It has long been my belief that one small change, done well and done repeatedly, is the secret to bringing about change to your health. Often the smallest changes bring about the biggest results – remember small hinges swing big doors.

It is when you join up all these dots that the magic happens! Fertility is so much more than eating the right foods and getting enough exercise. It is about creating a healthy, loving, and nurturing relationship with your body. Because when the penny finally drops and you realise that the food you have been eating, the hectic and stressful lifestyle you have been living is preventing you from having the life and the health or the family that you so desperately desire, that's when you take back control and that's when your dreams start to come true!

I can be contacted via my website: www.healthandharmony.info

Coming Home to Ourselves
by Sharon Fitzmaurice

My name is Sharon Fitzmaurice and I live in County Galway. I am married to John with two adult children, Matthew, and Scott. I am forty-nine years young and my work as a Holistic Wellness Coach/Therapist, Reiki Master, Mindfulness & Mediation Teacher, Speaker and Author have been as a result of my own deep personal healing journey.

On reading each chapter, I am sure that many of the therapist's stories resonated with you in some way, as they did with me. In truth, we are all not so different, we all feel deeply as we seek peace and fulfilment.

I believe that there is an opening in our hearts that allows life to move through us as we are all energetic beings in an energetic universe. In the movement through our life experiences, we learn, grow, and develop, finding a space within us that allows us to experience ourselves, not just as human beings but as spiritual beings. We grow to understand that our development from our first breath into this world to our last is a journey of discovery. How, where and who we travel with will be our greatest lessons in life.

As I sit and write this, it is July 2020 and we are coming to the end of weeks of restrictions due to the Corona Virus – Covid19. It shook the world and literally stopped us in our tracks. Schools closed, businesses pulled down the shutters and only essential services remained open. The fear that took over was palpable, there were so many questions being asked and no-one was able to give a definitive answer as to how it would affect you or your family and when we would be free to return to 'normal' life. We were fed fear-based stories daily and it became a time of anxiety for so many, not knowing what was going to happen. The 'not knowing' is a factor that I have often seen in people that creates anxiety and a lot of stress. We all seek answers, not just in a pandemic.

During the pandemic, it gave a lot of people time to reflect on their lives and for some, not having the distractions of a busy routine was a welcome gift to really look within. This is something I learned to do many years ago after contemplating suicide at the age of twenty-four. It was not just a spur of the moment decision; it was the accumulation of years of pain and trauma that had built up inside my mind and body, my spirit broken. For me at the time, I believed there was no other way to stop the pain that I was experiencing on a daily basis and had hidden from everyone. I lived with a mask of pretence and it had started to crack, revealing myself was one of the hardest things I ever did and I wasn't sure that I had the strength or courage to do it.

I wrote and published my story in my first book 'Someone please help me, So I did' in 2018 and that is when I realised that the past held no power over me anymore. It was like a weight had been lifted off my shoulders and I had been the one who chose to let it go. I didn't have to carry this burden of guilt, shame or bitterness any longer. It was now my choice to take responsibility for my own life and the take with me the lessons I had learned from the past in a positive and constructive way. In fact, revealing my vulnerability gave me the most strength as I realised more than ever with the response to my book that there are so many people out there suffering in silence. Many of my co-authors in this book are sharing their stories for the first time and for most it has been a very healing experience.

For those of you who have not read my story yet, I will give you a brief introduction into my life and how I came to be where I am today.

Growing up as a child was very traumatic as I was sexually abused for many years. I experienced domestic violence and for me, I believed this was what all families went through. Of course as I got older, I realised that not every family lived like this. Then the shame set in, which would develop into a lack of self-worth and lack of confidence. The anxiety I experienced was a daily fear of what was coming next — the waiting was sometimes worse than the actual abuse. I believed I must have deserved it in some way because I was a bad child or looked upon as not deserving of anything better. I could not tell my mother as I was afraid that she would not love me anymore and my abuser had made me believe that if I told anyone, I would be sent away to an institution. I believed it.

Even as I grew into young adulthood, I still carried the conditioning of my past and brought it into my relationships. I could not truly be honest about my hidden secrets as I believed no one would love me if I revealed my true self. I sought unconditional love, but if I could not give it to myself, how could I expect anyone else to either? At seventeen, I got pregnant and terrified of the consequences of this being found out and more shame being held in my mind. I travelled to the UK to get a termination, it was one of the most frightening experiences of my young adult life and in doing so, I saw first-hand the number of young girls and women travelling on a daily basis, mostly alone and with no support. You return home unable to share it with anyone and again, carrying shame and guilt. For some women they carried it to their graves. I went onto to get married at the age of twenty-two and it barely lasted a year. Again more shame to burden myself with now being separated. This is when I honestly believed that I was not worth loving and I silently berated myself daily about not being good enough and that I deserved all the pain in my life.

This led to the dark night of my soul when I considered suicide. For many people who have experienced suicide in their family or close circles, there is so much pain left behind, but from my own experience, I can only tell you how I felt at the time. I was so tired of the constant battle in my own mind, of pretending to others that I was fine. I felt as if I was losing any sense of self and becoming the pain that I was trying to push away and hide. I did not believe that I would be missed from this world. I had become a lesser version of myself. Even though I had so much love around me, I was not able to feel it. I had blocked myself from receiving or giving any real love to anyone, especially myself, so there was just a black void inside of my heart and my mind sank deeper and deeper into it every day.

Instead of leaving this world, I ended up awakening to a new awareness and understanding of wanting to live. This was the hardest choice I had ever made as it was down to me now to heal and reach out for support, in doing so I would have to reveal my pain and show others the shadows that I ran from. This was not an instant fix, but it was a second chance at life and now it was up to me how I wanted to live it. This is where the learning truly started for me.

In writing my story, first for myself as a daily healing journal/ diary, I found that I was so angry, bitter and resentful from what I had experienced in my childhood, I had a huge amount of blaming others going on in my head and my heart felt closed to forgiveness and in turn, I couldn't heal fully. I cried most days as I wrote and poured my heart out onto the pages, as each word flowed the tears flowed too. I felt like I was pulling from the deepest darkest spaces within me. There was so much fear in doing this as I was slowly allowing myself to feel everything that I had pushed aside so that I could function on a daily basis, but that is exactly what I was doing – functioning. I wasn't truly living.

I had heard the saying before *'leave the past in the past'* and thought this was a great way to not have to think about what had happened in my life, but suddenly as I wrote, I realised that I had to allow myself to feel the feelings, remember the memories and listen to my body as it wreathed in pain once again reliving the horrors of my childhood. I wanted to fight it and run away, but where was I running to, this was all inside of me and it would always be with me until I stopped, listened and truly honoured every feeling held within my being. I know from listening to my own clients now that they are still afraid of bringing up feelings connected to the memories surrounding those very painful times in their lives, but when they start to speak, their story starts to come out and they realise that they have held onto the pain and it has affected every other aspect of their life.

After letting go of the suicidal ideations as the answer to all my problems, I had made a choice to start living one day at a time — it literally was one minute at a time and felt like I was dragging my body to get to the next moment. During this time, I was practising mindfulness without realising it and it led me onto meditation where I allowed myself to sit quietly and not just experience the thoughts as they passed through my mind without getting attached to them or where the feelings were held in my body, but I allowed myself to go deeper into my heart. This was a space I had closed off for a long time and suddenly I was starting to find the strength to seek within its dark corridors, where I had shut the door on certain people and situations. I was ready to walk the darkest corridors of my life and step into the spaces where I needed to shine my own light.

Throughout my childhood, I had always been aware of people's energy and other energies present in our universe. I knew that they were not all of the physical but had no sense of what or who these energies could be. I learned later in my development that they were of the Spirit world, that they were my spiritual guides, angels and a lot of time my loved ones in Spirit trying to help me feel their love and support. Of course, I wasn't able to when I had closed myself off from seeing anything but fear. Once I started to show myself self-love, little by little, I started to experience their presence and guidance again. I know that we all come into this world with the awareness that we are more than just the physical body, but as human beings, we separate ourselves from believing we are part of the Divine and even after we leave this physical world, we still are present and connected by love.

I am not a religious person, but I do have faith. My faith is based on the goodness of others that help to transform the world into a place we all want to live in. Faith is trusting that even though you are struggling, you can and will get through whatever is going on for you right now. That is something I learned whilst growing up, somewhere deep inside of me there was a belief that I was being looked after on some other level. This I discovered to be true when I connected to my spiritual guides that had been with me all my life, but I couldn't connect to them when I was living in fear.

Around the physical body is an energy field called the aura. This aura is an energetic reflection of the physical body. It reflects the state of our physical health, mental and emotional well-being and it is the part of us that does not *die* with the physical body. Our consciousness remains as an energetic vibration in the Universe, so we do not forget who we are or who we knew. Knowing this has brought me peace, especially after my sister Bonnie passed away in 1998, and later in 2004, when I lost my little baby Annie. We still must grieve the physical loss of having that person in our life but knowing that they are still connected to us energetically through that strong bond of love is very comforting.

This practice of daily mindfulness and meditation led me to want to learn more as I, like many, had questioned my existence and why some of us go through the biggest challenges and others seem to float through life unaffected, so I dug deeper within myself and allowed myself to start trusting my intuition and listening to my inner guidance. I began to speak more positively to myself — this began the cycle of change for me. I had to practise what I was learning. I followed my gut and my heart with a great passion for learning more. The more I meditated, the more peace I found, the more peace I found, the more forgiveness I allowed, the more forgiveness I gave, the more space I made for love, the more love I experienced, the greater the joy in my life. One led to the other — I had to let go of the fear to experience the love.

Mindfulness is the practice of bringing your attention to the present moment without judgement, allowing yourself to experience everything in each moment and being fully present with it. It is called a practice for a reason as so many of us are either going back to the past or worrying about the future in our minds, we have forgotten the beauty of this moment. The practice of mindfulness allowed me to feel grounded in my physical body, to listen to my emotions without them overpowering me, it helped me to really see myself in the world without fear or worry. It helped me to really open my eyes to the world that I lived in and to myself, what I chose to focus on each day was my responsibility. If I continued to only see the negative in everyone and everything, this was a direct reflection of my own self-worth.

Although mindfulness helped me stay present and focused, I learned to go deeper within during my meditation practice with eyes closed and allowing myself to connect with the aspects of myself that were neither past or present, they were impermanent and this was where my interest in energy was aroused. I realised that as an energetic being, we are not bound to the physical body, but ever-changing. I always say that meditation saved my life, but it was more than that, meditation allowed me to explore aspects of myself that opened doors of hope, self-love, and inner strength. I have taken the most beautiful journeys inside my mind and heart and as I did, I released the heaviness I felt but somehow still feeling trapped within my physical body. I was freeing my mind from being a prisoner of the past and needed to do the same for my body.

Whilst re-training my mind to not react to the negative beliefs or conditioning that I had done for so long, I was now developing a new mindset in which I responded with compassion to those negative thoughts and feelings, allowing myself space to grow the more positive aspects of who I was. I am more than my past beliefs and experiences — I am who I believe I am. Whilst working on my mind on a daily basis, I still felt like my body carried a lot of trauma in my cells, even though I knew consciously that I was not a little girl fearing what would come next, sub-consciously I was triggered by certain things and my body responded by freezing or going into a state of panic. I wanted to learn how to heal all aspects of myself and so I discovered Reiki Energy Therapy. This is a non-evasive hands-on therapy that helps to clear and balance our energy – physically, mentally, emotionally, and spiritually.

As I continued to study more about how stress and trauma can affect our wellbeing, I understood why my body reacted to situations my unconscious mind perceived as a threat.

When something is too much for a person to handle, the nervous system goes into overload, stopping trauma from being processed. This overload stops the body in its instinctive fight or flight response causing the traumatic energy to be stored in the surrounding muscles, organs, and connective tissue. I call them invisible wounds. I got to feel every inner wound I held and realised they were open because I had not acknowledged them so they could heal.

Your body is made up of cells which are made up of atoms. You are an electric field of energy holding atoms together. Every atom has its own electric field which generates electrical signals and the human body creates electromagnetic fields. We all have electrical currents that run through every part of our human body; they are present in the nervous system, organs and cells, the electrical signals that trigger our heartbeat to travel throughout all the tissues of the body and can be detected anywhere in the body. When this electrical current flows through our body, an electromagnetic field is produced that reflects the nature of the current that created it. Electromagnetic fields are all around the body and around each of the organs, including the brain, heart, kidneys, liver, stomach etc. The heart has the strongest field. The fields around each of the organs pulse at different frequencies and stay within a specific frequency range when they are healthy but move out of this range when they are unbalanced.

The hands of the Reiki therapist produce a pulsing electromagnetic field when they are in the process of clearing or balancing your energy. When the therapist places their hands on or near the client in need of balancing, the electromagnetic field of the therapist's hands sweeps through a range of frequencies based on the needs of the part of the body being treated. The therapist induces a healthy electromagnetic field around an unhealthy organ, helping to induce a healthy state in the organ.

This is the scientific way to describe Reiki Energy Therapy, for me it is a deep but gentle healing that moves through layers of stress, pain, trauma, conditioning, and old belief systems to help you heal and come home to yourself. As a therapist, I work from my heart with compassion and non-judgement. I connect to the soul energy of my clients and allow it to show me what is right for each person at that moment. As an intuitive, I can feel or sense the area in which the energy of my client is unbalanced. I do not diagnose any medical conditions as I work on the energetic bodies to help bring them into alignment.

Reiki is a grounding energy and helps to bring your mind, body and soul into alignment with each other. In some cases of trauma, this is not always possible at first as the client has to acknowledge, accept and allow themselves to experience what they are holding onto, identify it (if possible) and choose what comes next. I am all for guiding the client and showing them in the present moment, what their energy is holding onto, but from there it is the client's choice in where we go next. I am helping to empower my clients to take responsibility for their own healing. In my experience, most physical dis-ease is a result of a mental and emotional issue that the client may be unaware of, but when we work together on finding the root cause, we start the healing process.

Not all clients are coming to me to heal issues from the past, some have lost their way in life and are trying to find the right direction to take next. Some of my clients just want time out and know that a relaxing reiki session keeps their energy balanced and immune system boosted. They see it as prevention rather than a cure. Like our cars, we all need to be fine-tuned every so often. We cannot run on empty and our bodies are the vehicles that give us the freedom to do so much. Many of my clients have been recommended to me by their doctors to work alongside conventional medicine. Amazingly, many of my clients are medical professionals themselves, and they too need support to be able to help their patients.

Other clients have issues from work, friends, family members that are out of their control, but nonetheless still affects them on some level. I understand these feelings as I have a big family and there is always something going on for the people I care about. I know now that I cannot fix or sort out their problems and learning to step back is a big one for me! This is especially true when it comes to our children. My children are young adults now, but I still want to nurture and support them as much as I can, sometimes they don't want that and as a mother I have to learn to respect their space and freedom. As a therapist, I must respect that they may not want my help with issues they are facing as we are too emotionally involved and that it is better to guide them to someone else who comes with no attachments. My best advice to all parents is just keep letting your kids know that you are there for them no matter what. Try not to let your fears and worries become a part of your child's anxieties.

As a therapist, I use every skill and my life experience to provide the client with as much information as possible in each session to allow them to understand that in opening our awareness of understanding what is going on for us may be as a result of something that happened in the past and we react to it the same way we always did. In changing the way we look at ourselves, we change how we respond to our needs as they arise.

I have worked with people of all ages, cultures, backgrounds and professions. When it comes down to it we are all looking for the answer to our problems, we are quick to focus on the problem, but may not always be aware of the many options that are available to us. Instead of asking my client *"What is wrong"*, I ask *"How do you want to feel?"* Many clients may have trouble getting in touch with their feelings as they are not fully present in their body. Our bodies record each painful experience in our lives, big or small. Pushing away or denying our feelings is our learned behaviour and we learned to not be present in our bodies so as not to have to deal with what we were experiencing or feeling. We repeat this behaviour or pattern every time we experience something that we feel is threatening us in some way. When we do not allow ourselves to feel, our energy becomes ungrounded and fragmented.

As I work with any of my clients, their innermost fears and dreams start to come to the surface; with each one, there is a choice to hold on or let it go. Sometimes there is a fear of if *"I let this old story go, who will I be without it?"* That is where the real healing starts, and you start to transform. Accepting that the old story is no longer you, but you are here because of it. Acknowledging the aspects your story taught you will help you to take ownership of your present life and move forward into your future life.

As part of my role as a therapist and teacher in mindfulness, meditation and reiki energy therapy, I also trained in Clinical Hypnotherapy and Psychotherapy, and this happened again due to the passion I have for learning and discovering more ways in which I could firstly help myself and, in turn, others. If we continue to do things the same way we always did, we are not learning. I am all for learning something new and sharing it with others as much as possible, that is what knowledge is for — to be shared. When learning, you are forming new connections in your brain. You may have heard of Neuroplasticity, the brain's ability to reorganise itself by forming new neural connections throughout life. The brain is constantly changing and creating new pathways as a reaction to thoughts, emotions, and experiences.

Our brains contain about one billion neurons. Every time you learn a new skill, have a new experience, think a new thought, you change your brain. If you keep thinking the same thoughts and repeat the same behaviour, you keep firing the same neural patterns. You create automatic behaviours and responses to everything that happens in your life. If the behaviours are positive, you will see positive changes in your life. The same goes for negative behaviours. The brain does not make a distinction between imagined and real. The mind believes only what we tell it.

You use your mind every day, every minute to heal you or to harm you. Your thinking is reflected in your body. Your body reacts to your thoughts. Becoming more aware of your self-talk is the first step in recognising what story you tell yourself or others. If your story is one of being a victim and feeling powerless in your own life, it is time to change the narrative.

By repeating the new thoughts and behaviours, you will create new neural pathways. You will literally change your brain as the brain will delete the neural connections, that are no longer needed. In your life, if you want to experience happiness, confidence, calmness, creativity, or resilience, you learn to re-shape your mind with your thoughts, that reflect those qualities.

Identifying where you want change in your life, firstly means understanding how your mind and body work and then making daily changes to create the life you genuinely want. It sounds easy, but in fact, our brain is wired to respond to negativity. It is called the negativity bias. Our brain is wired according to the experiences we have in our early years and to the environment we have grown up in. That is why everyone's brain is different. We learn how to think, speak, and react from those around us. If this was mostly negative for you, then it will reflect in your thoughts, words, and actions. It has a huge impact on how your think, how your brain functions and even on your physical, mental, and emotional health. This has a huge impact on our lives, our relationships and on our society.

Our experiences in how we see ourselves and the world are a direct result of our learning in childhood, but I am proof that we can change the negative bias in our brains and go on to live a full and happy life by learning that daily changes, self-awareness, personal development and being completely honest with yourself can help you reconnect with the person you choose to be. It all comes down to your choices — no matter what your circumstances are.

For me, it starts with a thought in your mind to change, then a belief that you can create the change. As a person that believed she was not worthy of much, I learned to develop the belief that I could do anything I set my mind to. I am not talking about material wealth, as that is fleeting. I set my mind to developing personally and then professionally, to help others to help themselves. As you are teaching or guiding others, you are also learning from their experiences and that brings new insights into your awareness. It all happens when you are truly present with a person and listening, not just to their words, but to the energy that emits from them. This is where our intuitive abilities are developed. We are listening with all our senses and really seeing, hearing, and feeling the person. When you truly see a person, you see their past, present and future within them. This is the light that guides me as a therapist and if I listen to this, I can help guide them to follow their own light. That light is their soul.

I had found myself in a place of darkness that enveloped and shrouded me from fully experiencing life because of my fears and beliefs when I connected to the light within. I had to learn to think, speak and act in a way that was new to me. There were days in which I allowed myself to slip silently into that dark lonely place, but with everything I have learned, I would connect to my light and remind myself that when you bring the light into the darkness it's not so scary, it has much to teach us and its where our healing happens.

I honour the feelings and thoughts as they arise. I speak them truthfully now to the ones that I trust and love me unconditionally. I am not afraid to show my vulnerability and know that by expressing how I feel gives me strength and in that strength, I have nothing to hide from or fear as I am true to myself and others. On many occasions, having been asked to speak at different events, my first thought would be the negative thought *"Why would they ask me. I can't do that!"*, this is a constant reminder to me that my first reaction is a fearful one, to run away from anything that is outside of my comfort zone. So fully aware of its presence, I remind myself and my mind that you were asked because you have much to say on this topic, people want you to share your experiences for a reason and every time you step up, you are helping another person. With that, I respond with an incredibly grateful yes to all invitations and start preparing for the event.

We can't always be prepared for every event in life, but if we practice on a daily basis, focusing our attention and actions on what is bringing us to a safer and more loving place within ourselves and in our environment, we can deal with the challenges that occur in our personal and professional lives with a more practical and positive response. This is what I share with all participants in my workshops, reiki and mindfulness trainings, retreats and when I am speaking to groups or organisations. Each day is an opportunity for us to expand our awareness into all that we want to be. I am still learning and by sharing this book, we are not only expanding your awareness but by sharing the information with you, we are helping you choose what you feel may be right to help your wellbeing.

Over the years, I have been presented with situations that challenged me to the fullest. When I reflect on them now, I know that they were not happening to me, but like you, it took me time to come back to myself and focus on what is important. Whether it is something that you face, or it is a family member or friend, know that you falling to pieces is not going to make the situation any better. We find a place within ourselves and in it, we ask ourselves the important questions, *"How can I help in this situation?"* or *"Do I take a step back?"*

An example is when my mother was diagnosed with cancer last year and suddenly, we were faced with the possibility of losing her. My youngest son is going through a huge transition in his life for the past year and at times, I feel helpless. We first face our own pain within the situation, this is where empathy comes into play, you feel the suffering of the other person, but if you continue to suffer, you are then unable to help them, so we come to a place of compassion for ourselves and for them. When we face the fear of not knowing how to help them, we can be there to fully support them, even if we do not really have a clue how to do that. I just focus on the love I have for them with my every thought and sometimes, I scream into my pillow!

For anyone that is supporting someone in their lives that is unwell in any way, you can only do your best, but you must look after yourself too. You cannot look after anyone else if you do not look after yourself first. Seek advice from other people who are going through a similar situation and admit to yourself when you need support.

I feel an emotion rising to the surface and know this to be joy. I am truly blessed with so much love and light in my life right now, my wonderful husband John who has been the external light that seeks the light in me to show itself fully and wholeheartedly. My 'big kids' Matthew and Scott are my reason for thriving; I would like them to see their mother with all her imperfections and owning each one knowing that we don't have to be the perfect parent. If we show ourselves love and compassion, we can be better parents to our children. Allowing them space to grow and develop into who they want to be. I am so proud of them both and know that a little spark of me resides inside their energy and that even when I have long passed from this world, I will always be in their hearts. A practical and compassionate book for all parents with anxious children is '*Love In, Love Out*' by Dr. Malie Coyne.

I am profoundly grateful for the wonderful therapists who collaborated in this book with me and honoured to share it with you in the hope that it will also help Galway Simon Community to do more in preventing homelessness in our communities. When asked why I am a long-time supporter of Galway Simon's work, I tell people how I felt as a child and young adult surviving week to week in rented accommodation and not knowing if we would have enough food to eat, if the rent was paid. There are many people out there in the same situation even now in 2020. Families are struggling to pay rent and mortgages and sometimes go without heat or food to keep a roof over their head. There are many families living in hotels and shelters, not knowing if they will ever have a space to call their own. Homelessness affects so many people in Ireland right now with increasing rents and the shortage of affordable housing. This all leads to increased stress which has a knock-on effect on our wellbeing. Many young people must leave their family homes due to issues beyond their control. I have seen first-hand the work and support of Galway Simon in helping people stay in education and provide them with a place to call their home leading to independent living.

Home is not where you are from. It is where you find light when all grows dark.

My parting message to all who are reading this book is to be more compassionate and understanding of yourself and others.

We are only passing through this world and learning from each other. Wherever you are in your life right now, it is okay — know that all changes cannot be made overnight and taking just one step towards the life you want to live is going to be the start of awakening your wellbeing. We all feel alone at times and feel that no-one will understand what we have or are going through, but I promise you, there is always someone out there who does. Healing is not about making your pain disappear; it is allowing your hurt and struggles to be seen, felt, and heard. It starts with acknowledging how you feel. Our emotions are warning signals that tell us to pay attention to how we are reacting to a person or situation. Accept that connecting to the sadness and fear is hard, but it is much harder trying to hide it. You deserve to be seen, heard, and loved. Think about all that you are, instead of all that you are not.

May you be well
May you be happy
May you find peace

For now, start with looking within, developing the relationship you have with yourself will help you navigate your journey.

The butterfly is proof that you can go through a whole lot of darkness and still become something beautiful

A simple practice to get your started

Close your eyes and take a deep breath into your heart, hold for a moment, and breathe out fully, letting go of anything that feels heavy in your mind or body.

1. Acknowledge how you feel, name the feeling, where is it held in your body?
2. Breathe into that feeling without judgement or criticism, now breathe into it x 5 times

3. What lays beneath that feeling? This is where you learn the most.
4. Place your hands on your heart and say *"I am doing my best."*
5. Find one thing to be grateful for each day.
6. Smile more.
7. Take 10 minutes each day to write or journal – seeing it as energetically letting go of anything that is bothering you and allowing yourself to express your emotions.
8. Create an affirmation or mantra to repeat to yourself in times of doubt or fear.
   "My mind is quiet, still and clear" or *"I am kind to myself and others."*
9. Sing out loud to your favourite song – dance along! (My favourite!)
10. Take a walk or spend time in nature every day.
11. Meditate a little each day – simply start with observing your breath. (I have free guided meditations on YouTube to get you started.)
12. Volunteer – helping others has a huge impact on our wellbeing.
13. Plan something special for yourself every week — it does not have to cost money!

- Meet a friend for a walk – go somewhere new each week
- Have a bath – use Epsom salts for detox or lavender to relax.
- Read a book – join a book club
- Take a photo of one thing that made you smile each week – create an album
- Keep a gratitude journal. *(I have one available on my website to get you started.)*

Do Less Of:
Comparing your progress to others
Saying yes to everything
Focusing on what you do not have
Trying to get rid of thoughts
Judging yourself for feeling bad

Do More Of:
Praising yourself for the little things
Saying NO without having to say why
Grateful for what you do have
 Notice thoughts coming and going
Celebrate when you feel good

Website
www.sharonfitzmauricemindfulness.com
Free Guided Meditations
www.youtube.com/user/safitzm
www.insightimer.com/sharonfitzmaurice
Facebook
Awaken Your Potential with Sharon Fitzmaurice
Instagram @sharonfitzmaurice_wellbeing

Please Review

Dear Reader,

Thank you for taking the time to read this book. If you found it helpful, please help spread the message to others who may be seeking this information. Please visit Amazon, or the platform where you purchased this book to write a review. A review can also be left on Goodreads. This matters because most potential readers first judge a book by what others have to say. An honest review would be most appreciated.

The proceeds from the sale of this book is going towards funding a very worthy cause; namely Galway Simon Community.

Thanking you for your support and generosity.

CPSIA information can be obtained
at www.ICGtesting.com
Printed in the USA
LVHW080252221020
669488LV00018B/1985